2014

The Year Book of PLASTIC AND AESTHETIC SURGERY™

Editor-in-Chief

Stephen H. Miller, MD, MPH

Clinical Professor of Surgery and Family Medicine (non-salaried), University of California San Diego, San Diego, California

ELSEVIER
MOSBY

ELSEVIER
MOSBY

VP Global Medical Reference: Mary E. Gatsch
Editor: Joanne C. Husovski
Production Manager, Electronic Year Books: Donna M. Skelton
Electronic Article Manager: Mike Sheets
Illustrations and Permissions Coordinator: Dawn Vohsen

2014 EDITION

Composition by TNQ Books and Journals Pvt Ltd, India

Editorial Office:
Elsevier
1600 John F. Kennedy Blvd.
Suite 1800
Philadelphia, PA 19103-2899

International Standard Serial Number: 1535-1513
International Standard Book Number: 978-0-323-26483-9

Printed and bound by CPI Group (UK) Ltd, Croydon, CR0 4YY

Transferred to digital print 2013

Editorial Board

Table of Contents

Journals Represented

Journals represented in this YEAR BOOK are listed below.

Aesthetic Plastic Surgery
Aesthetic Surgery Journal
American Journal of Otolaryngology
Annals of Plastic Surgery
Annals of Thoracic Surgery
Archives of Facial Plastic Surgery
British Journal of Surgery
Clinical Orthopaedics and Related Research
Dermatologic Surgery
Dermatology
European Journal of Plastic Surgery
Journal of Bone and Joint Surgery (American)
Journal of Clinical Periodontology
Journal of Drugs in Dermatology
Journal of Hand Surgery
Journal of Oral and Maxillofacial Surgery
Journal of Plastic, Reconstructive & Aesthetic Surgery
Journal of Reconstructive Microsurgery
Journal of Surgical Research
Journal of the American Academy of Dermatology
Journal of the European Academy of Dermatology & Venereology
Laryngoscope
Microsurgery
Orthopedics
Plastic and Reconstructive Surgery
Proceedings of the National Academy of Sciences of the United States of America

STANDARD ABBREVIATIONS

The following terms are abbreviated in this edition: acquired immunodeficiency syndrome (AIDS), cardiopulmonary resuscitation (CPR), central nervous system (CNS), cerebrospinal fluid (CSF), computed tomography (CT), deoxyribonucleic acid (DNA), electrocardiography (ECG), health maintenance organization (HMO), human immunodeficiency virus (HIV), intensive care unit (ICU), intramuscular (IM), intravenous (IV), magnetic resonance (MR) imaging (MRI), ribonucleic acid (RNA), ultrasound (US), and ultraviolet (UV).

NOTE

The YEAR BOOK OF PLASTIC AND AESTHETIC SURGERY is a literature survey service providing abstracts of articles published in the professional literature. Every effort is made to assure the accuracy of the information presented in these pages. Neither the editors nor the publisher of the YEAR BOOK OF PLASTIC AND AESTHETIC SURGERY can be responsible for errors in the original materials. The editors' comments are their own opinions. Mention of specific products within this publication does not constitute endorsement.

To facilitate the use of the YEAR BOOK OF PLASTIC AND AESTHETIC SURGERY as a reference tool, all illustrations and tables included in this publication are now identified as they appear in the original article. This change is meant to help the reader recognize that any illustration or table appearing in the YEAR BOOK OF PLASTIC AND AESTHETIC SURGERY may be only one of many in the original article. For this reason, figure and table numbers will often appear to be out of sequence within the YEAR BOOK OF PLASTIC AND AESTHETIC SURGERY.

Introduction

Once again, our publishers have decided to offer the YEAR BOOK OF PLASTIC AND AESTHETIC SURGERY on both electronic and hard copy. Whether or not this will continue in the future is uncertain at this time.

For those who keep track of the comings and goings of the Associate Editors, you will notice a much smaller group participating in this year's edition. We would like to acknowledge, with appreciation, the past fine efforts of Drs Amanda Gosman, James Boehmler, Robert Ruberg, and Roger Salisbury.

I am especially grateful to the two Associate Editors, Karol Gutowski and David Smith, who have once again done a fine job in selecting and critiquing the articles. In some instances, as in past years, more than one editor has selected and critiqued the same article. I believe this is worthwhile, as it provides the reader with differing viewpoints.

Thank you to Joanne Husovski, Senior Clinic Editor with Elsevier, who aided our efforts this year.

Stephen H. Miller, MD, MPH

1 Congenital

Cleft Lip and Palate

Constructing the Philtral Column in the Secondary Cleft Lip Deformity: Utilizing the Palmaris Longus Graft

Lim AA, Allam KA, Taneja R, et al (Naval Med Ctr, Portsmouth, VA; Sohag Univ Hosp, Egypt; Fortis Flt. Lt. Rajan Dhali Hosp, New Delhi, India; et al)

Ann Plast Surg 70:296-300, 2013

Background.—The philtrum and the Cupid's bow are the most prominent features of the upper lip and are crucial for normal appearance. Unfortunately, projection of the philtral column is a common deficiency of the repaired cleft lip. Although a multitude of methods for constructing the philtral dimple and ridge have been described, no single procedure has achieved complete satisfactory results. The authors describe their technique for construction of the philtral column using palmaris longus tendon.

Methods.—Between 1998 and 2009, a retrospective study was performed for identifying patients with depression of the philtral scar following cleft lip repair. Pre- and postoperative photographs were taken with at least 6 months follow-up. Postoperative patient satisfaction and occurrence of complications are reported.

Results.—In all, 17 patients who developed depression of the philtral ridge following cleft lip repair underwent philtral reconstruction utilizing palmaris longus tendon grafts by the senior author (H.K.K.). At the time of surgery, average age for 11 females and 6 males was 18.5 years. The follow-up period ranged from 6 to 126 months, with an average of 42.3 months. In the early postoperative period, 2 complications in the form of graft exposure occurred. However, both cases were successfully managed with preservation of the graft. All patients were satisfied with their long-term results, and none required further surgery.

Conclusions.—The use of palmaris longus tendon graft is an effective, reproducible, and safe method by which to construct the philtral column in the secondary cleft lip deformity (Fig 7).

▶ Successful secondary correction of a depressed and scarred philtral ridge after cleft lip repair is difficult to achieve. The authors present a useful, relatively simple, and minimally invasive technique, which, in their experience, has provided good results. They utilize a segment of the palmaris longus tendon folded onto itself

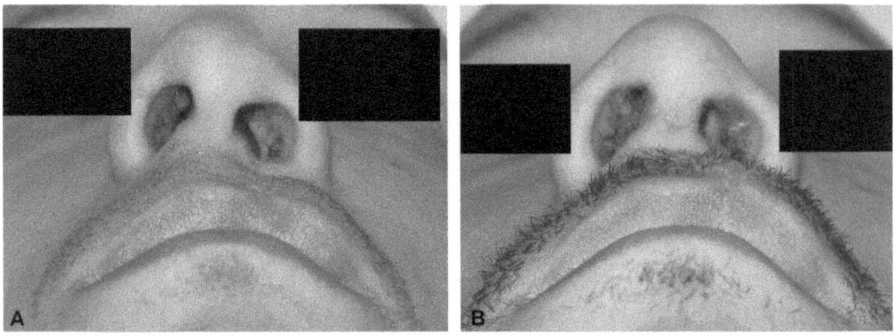

FIGURE 7.—A, preoperative photograph. B, postoperative photograph taken 9 months after palmaris graft to left philtrum and 6 months after rhinoplasty. (Reprinted from Lim AA, Allam KA, Taneja R, et al. Constructing the philtral column in the secondary cleft lip deformity: utilizing the palmaris longus graft. *Ann Plast Surg*. 2013;70:296-300, with permission from Lippincott Williams & Wilkins.)

to create a thicker graft than would be possible with a single layer on the tendon. Apparently, in those with long-term follow-up, the results remain satisfactory. Several concerns need to be addressed, not the least of which are better standardization of the photography used to measure and record the results and some way to objectify those results. Additionally, one might consider the use of nearby temporalis fascia, especially those lacking a palmaris tendon, as it is also easily accessible and in the same operative field as the lip while producing a scar more easily hidden than one on the wrist. I have found temporalis fascia to be an excellent source of autologous filler in several procedures.

S. H. Miller, MD

Congenital

Thumb Hypoplasia

Soldado F, Zlotolow DA, Kozin SH (Universitat Autonoma de Barcelona, Spain; Shriners Hosp for Children, Philadelphia, PA)
J Hand Surg 38A:1435-1444, 2013

Thumb hypoplasia, congenital underdevelopment of the thumb, can range from a slight decrease in thumb size to complete absence of the thumb. As part of the radial longitudinal deficiency spectrum, other organ systems may be affected as well. Hence, the global health of the child should be addressed before focusing on the thumb. The decision of whether to reconstruct the existing thumb or to ablate the thumb and perform a pollicization of the index finger hinges primarily on the examination of trapeziometacarpal joint stability. Ultrasound imaging may play a role in decision making in borderline cases. The ultimate goal of surgical treatment is to provide a stable and functional thumb.

▶ The authors present a current-concepts review of thumb hypoplasia. This underdevelopment of the thumb can range from a slight decrease in thumb size to complete absence of the thumb. The decision of whether to reconstruct the existing thumb or to ablate the thumb and do a pollicization of the index finger hinges primarily on the examination of trapeziometacarpal joint stability. This is a superb review on all aspects of thumb hypoplasia and a must-read for anyone doing congenital hand surgery. For the occasional surgeon, this is a wonderful update.

D. J. Smith, Jr, MD

2 Neoplastic, Inflammatory, and Degenerative Conditions

Trunk, Genitalia, and Extremities

A Comparative Study of Thoracoscopic Sympathicotomy Versus Local Surgical Treatment for Axillary Hyperhidrosis

Heidemann E, Licht PB (Odense Univ Hosp, Denmark)

Ann Thorac Surg 95:264-268, 2013

Background.—Axillary hyperhidrosis affects approximately 1.4% of the population. Medical management is often frustrating, and the response generally transient. Surgical methods include thoracoscopic sympathectomy or sympathicotomy and local axillary surgery such as suction-curettage or en-bloc skin resection. Many case series with retrospective follow-up are available in the literature, but no comparative studies between surgical techniques have been published.

Methods.—During a 9-year period, two groups of consecutive patients with isolated axillary hyperhidrosis underwent thoracoscopic sympathicotomy ($n = 49$) or local axillary surgery ($n = 47$) at the same university hospital, depending on referral or preference. Patients received identical questionnaires to investigate local effect and side effects after surgery.

Results.—Questionnaires were returned by 92% after a median of 26 months, with no significant difference between the two groups. Local effect was significantly better after axillary surgery compared with sympathicotomy ($p < 0.001$), but mild recurrent axillary symptoms were significantly more frequent after axillary surgery (51% versus 5%, $p < 0.001$). Compensatory and gustatory sweating were significantly more frequent after sympathicotomy (84% versus 25%, $p < 0.001$; and 54% versus 26%, $p = 0.01$, respectively).

Conclusions.—Outcome after surgery for isolated axillary hyperhidrosis was significantly better after local surgical treatment compared with sympathicotomy. Local effect was better and side effects fewer, but milder recurrent symptoms were more frequent. Compensatory sweating also occurs after local axillary surgery and has not been reported before. Our results suggest that local axillary surgery is preferable for isolated axillary hyperhidrosis and that R2-R3 or R2-R4 sympathicotomy should be discouraged. Sympathicotomy should only be considered for patients who have additional palmar hyperhidrosis.

▶ Axillary hyperhidrosis has many treatment options and frequently is not covered by health insurance plans. There is more evidence that sympathectomy does not provide good long-term results and that local treatment may be better (and less expensive). In this patient series, en-bloc axillary skin resection and axillary suction curettage were the local axillary surgery procedures. Both of these techniques can be done by plastic surgeons for their patients who decline treatment with botulinum toxin injections.

K. A. Gutowski, MD

Differences between objective efficacy and perceived efficacy in patients with palmar hyperhidrosis treated with either botulinum toxin or endoscopic thoracic sympathectomy

Álvarez MA, Ruano J, Gómez FJ, et al (Reina Sofia Univ Hosp, Cordoba, Spain)

J Eur Acad Dermatol Venereol 27:e282-e288, 2013

Background.—Moderate to severe palmar hyperhidrosis can disturb people's work and social and emotional lives. Botulinum toxin and sympathectomy are currently considered the most effective treatment options but few studies have analysed the concordance between efficacy and patient satisfaction in comparisons of these two types of treatments.

Objective.—To assess the relation between efficacy and the satisfaction of patients with palmar hyperhidrosis treated with either botulinum toxin or endoscopic thoracic sympathectomy.

Material and Methods.—This retrospective, observational study included all patients treated with either botulinum toxin or endoscopic thoracic sympathectomy in a single reference hospital in 2005–2010. Information was obtained from computerized medical records and a telephone survey about patients' educational and socio-economic level, awareness of treatment options, pre- and post-treatment severity of palmar hyperhidrosis, satisfaction and associated side effects. Predictors of efficacy and patient satisfaction with each treatment were analysed with ordinal and multinomial logistic regression models.

Results.—Patients who underwent sympathectomy had more severe palmar hyperhidrosis but efficacy and patient satisfaction were greater compared with patients given botulinum toxin. The severity of the compensatory palmar hyperhidrosis was predictive of less satisfaction after sympathectomy. In the group treated with botulinum toxin, low socio-economic status, lack of information about treatment options, fewer sessions and a shorter anhidrotic effect were associated with less satisfaction.

Conclusion.—In studies of expectations regarding the outcome of palmar hyperhidrosis treatment, doctors should consider the factors that determine patient satisfaction in relation to the treatment options.

▶ Unlike treatment for axillary hyperhidrosis, endoscopic sympathectomy may be a good choice for severe palmar hyperhidrosis and appears to provide better patient satisfaction than botulinum toxin injections. For milder cases, botulinum toxin should be considered first.

K. A. Gutowski, MD

The comparative effectiveness of suction-curettage and onabotulinumtoxin-A injections for the treatment of primary focal axillary hyperhidrosis: A randomized control trial

Ibrahim O, Kakar R, Bolotin D, et al (Northwestern Univ, Chicago, IL; et al)
J Am Acad Dermatol 69:88-95, 2013

Background.—Botulinum toxin injections and suction-curettage have been separately shown to be effective in treating axillary hyperhidrosis but have not been compared in the same patients.

Objective.—We sought to compare effectiveness of suction-curettage versus neurotoxin for the treatment of axillary hyperhidrosis.

Methods.—Each of 20 patients was randomized to receive toxin injections to one axilla and suction-curettage to the contralateral axilla. The primary outcome measure was reduction of sweat rate measured by gravimetry, and the secondary measure was quality of life as measured by a patient-directed questionnaire.

Results.—At 3 months posttreatment, toxin injections decreased baseline resting sweat production by 72.1% versus 60.4% (P =.29) for suction-curettage, and baseline exercise-induced sweat production by 73.8% versus 58.8% (P =.10). When patients were stratified into the categories of light and heavy sweaters, there was a difference among heavy sweaters, with exercise-induced sweat production lower by 10.48 mg/min or 34.3% (P =.0025) at toxin-treated sites. Compared with suction-curettage, toxin also resulted in greater improvements in quality of life by 0.80 points (P =.0002) and 0.90 points (P =.0017) at 3 and 6 months posttreatment, respectively, as measured by the patient questionnaire.

Limitations.—The follow-up period was limited to 6 months.

Conclusions.—By objective measures 3 months after treatment, neurotoxin injections are nominally more effective than suction-curettage in all cases, and markedly more effective in heavy sweaters. Patients have a very significant preference for neurotoxin injections at 3 months, and this is maintained at 6 months.

▶ This study supports the use of botulinum toxin injections over suction-assisted curettage for axillary hyperhidrosis. However, some patients may not favor the repeated cost and treatments of botulinum toxin, and, for them, curettage may be a better choice. Patients should know, however, that although the effects of suction-assisted curettage have been shown to typically last more than 1 year, long-term data are lacking, and some patients do relapse after a few years. Also, cases of compensatory palmar hyperhidrosis have been reported (which can be treated by endoscopic sympathectomy). Surgical excision of axillary skin may be a better option but does result in more visible scars. New technologies, such as microwave thermolysis or high-frequency ultrasound scan, may also be considered, but long-term comparative studies have not been done.

K. A. Gutowski, MD

3 Hand and Upper Extremity

General

What's New in Hand Surgery
Amadio PC (Mayo Clinic, Rochester, MN)
J Bone Joint Surg Am 94:569-573, 2012

Background.—The material presented at the 2011 annual meetings of the American Society for Surgery of the Hand (ASSH), the American Association for Hand Surgery (AAHS), and the American Academy of Orthopaedic Surgeons (AAOS) and selected articles in the area of hand surgery were reviewed. Updates were noted in skeletal trauma, tendon injury, replantation and microsurgery, other vascular problems, arthritis, Dupuytren contracture, Kienböck disease, and cost-effectiveness in hand surgery.

Updates.—With respect to skeletal trauma, updates were found in the management of distal radial fracture, bone quality and bone density in osteoporosis screening, intercarpal ligament and cartilage injuries, carpal tunnel release during volar plating of the distal part of the radius, use of simple distal pole excision for posttraumatic arthritis secondary to scaphoid nonunion, scaphoid fractures, and scapholunate injuries. Tendon injury management may be altered by the ability to practice surgical techniques in benchtop simulations and by active mobilization after repair. Access to replantation services is highly inconsistent and offers challenges to many communities. Toe-to-hand transfer techniques all appear to have comparable outcomes.

Raynaud phenomenon may respond to botulinum toxin type A treatment, but sodium hyaluronate, while safe for arthritis of the thumb, appears ineffective. Implants are similarly ineffective as replacements for the base of the thumb metacarpal in terms of strength and motion. Proximal interphalangeal joint arthroplasty remains problematic. Total wrist arthroplasty with an implant produces high patient satisfaction but not always clinically acceptable results. Collagenase for Dupuytren contracture and other minimally invasive approaches appear to be associated with lower rates of recurrence at the metacarpophalangeal joints than at the proximal interphalangeal joints. However, patients appear to be unconcerned with the degree of contracture, which does not correlate strongly with the degree of functional impairment. Interestingly, hand surgeons cannot agree on the radiographic appearance of Kienböck disease, even with their own previous assessments.

It was pointed out that professionals should be aware of the effectiveness of treatments but also of the cost to patients. Formal hand therapy programs often cost more but are no more effective than informal rehabilitation instructions from the surgeon. Repair of hand fractures in a minor surgical suite appears to be safe and effective and costs much less than care delivered in an operating room. Also, field sterility is sufficient for carpal tunnel surgery, saves time and money, and cuts down on waste. Similar findings were related to antibiotics and pain medications, both of which tend to be overly prescribed. Patients end up with extra medication, which poses a risk for inappropriate use.

Conclusions.—Many areas were updated in the annual meetings of the ASSH, AAHS, and AAOS and in hand surgery articles published between August 2010 and July 2011. Keeping abreast of these changes will have an impact on care.

▶ The author reviews material presented at the 2011 annual meetings of the American Society for Surgery of the Hand, American Association for Hand Surgery, and the American Academy of Orthopedic Surgeons as well as articles published in the field of hand surgery (other than those published in *The Journal of Bone & Joint Surgery*) between August 2010 and July 2011. This is an excellent overview for those wanting to stay current in hand surgery but whose practice is not primarily focused in that area.

D. J. Smith, Jr, MD

Program Director Opinions of Core Competencies in Hand Surgery Training: Analysis of Differences between Plastic and Orthopedic Surgery Accredited Programs

Sears ED, Larson BP, Chung KC (Univ of Michigan Health System, Ann Arbor; Veterans Administration Health System, Ann Arbor, MI)

Plast Reconstr Surg 131:582-590, 2013

Background.—The authors' aim was to conduct a national survey of hand surgery fellowship program directors to determine differences of opinions of essential components of hand surgery training between program directors from plastic and orthopedic surgery programs.

Methods.—The authors performed a Web-based survey of 74 program directors from all Accreditation Council for Graduate Medical Education–accredited hand surgery fellowship programs to determine components that are essential for hand surgery training. The survey included assessment of nine general areas of practice, 97 knowledge topics, and 172 procedures. Twenty-seven scales of related survey items were created to determine differences between specialty groups based on clinical themes.

Results.—An 84 percent response rate was achieved, including 49 orthopedic and 12 plastic surgery program directors. There were significant differences in mean responses between the specialty groups in 11 of 27 scales. Only one scale, forearm fractures, contained items with a significantly stronger preference for essential rating among orthopedic surgeons. The other 10 scales contained items with a significantly higher preference for essential rating among plastic surgeons, most of which related to soft-tissue injury and reconstruction. The burn scale had the greatest discrepancy in opinion of essential ratings between the groups, followed by pedicled and free tissue transfer, and amputation and fingertip injuries.

Conclusions.—Despite being united under the subspecialty of hand surgery, program directors tend to emphasize clinical areas that are stressed in their respective primary disciplines. These differences promote the advantage of programs that provide exposure to both plastic surgery–trained and orthopedic surgery–trained hand surgeons.

▶ These authors conducted a national survey of hand surgery fellowship program directors to determine the differences of opinions of essential components of hand surgery training between program directors from plastic and orthopedic surgery programs. Not surprisingly, program directors tend to emphasize clinical areas that are stressed in their respective primary disciplines. These differences highlight one of the many challenges in achieving competency-based training in hand surgery. This emphasizes the advantages of programs providing exposure to both plastic surgery–trained and orthopedic surgery–trained hand surgeons. Otherwise, the isolated specialty training will be maintained and the limitation of experience compounded.

D. J. Smith, Jr, MD

The Quality of Systematic Reviews in Hand Surgery: An Analysis Using AMSTAR

Momeni A, Lee GK, Talley JR (Stanford Univ Med Ctr, Palo Alto, CA)

Plast Reconstr Surg 131:831-837, 2013

Background.—Systematic reviews constitute the top of the "level-of-evidence pyramid." Despite their strengths, they have been found to be of varying quality, thus raising concerns about their validity and role in influencing clinical practice. In the present study, a quality analysis of systematic reviews with a focus on hand surgery was performed.

Methods.—A PubMed search was performed to identify all systematic reviews published up to and including December of 2011 in eight surgical journals. Two authors independently reviewed the literature and extracted data from included reviews. Discrepancies were resolved by consensus. Quality assessment was performed using AMSTAR.

Results.—The initial search retrieved 687 articles. After screening titles and abstracts, 635 articles were excluded. Full-text review of the remaining

52 articles resulted in further exclusion of 10 articles, leaving 42 systematic reviews for final analysis. A significant increase in the number of published systematic reviews over time was noted ($p = 0.04$), with the majority of systematic reviews being published in *The Journal of Hand Surgery* ($n = 19$) and *Plastic and Reconstructive Surgery* ($n = 12$). Although a significant improvement in the quality of systematic reviews was noted over time ($p = 0.01$), a median AMSTAR score of 7 indicated the bulk of reviews to be of fair to good quality.

Conclusions.—The trend to publish more systematic reviews in hand surgery is paralleled by an increase in the quality of systematic reviews. Nonetheless, increased efforts are indicated to further improve the quality of systematic reviews in hand surgery.

▶ Systematic reviews constitute the top of the level-of-evidence pyramid. Despite their strengths, systematic reviews have been found to be of varying quality, thus raising concerns about their validity and role in influencing clinical practice. These authors note that the trend to publish more systematic reviews on hand surgery is paralleled by an increase in the quality of systematic reviews. Still, overall, the quality remains average. Editors must assume more responsibility when publishing systematic reviews. Conversely, we, the readers, must become more critical and not take systematic reviews as gospel.

D. J. Smith, Jr, MD

Guidelines for Ethical and Professional Use of Social Media in a Hand Surgery Practice

Lifchez SD, McKee DM, Raven RB III, et al (Johns Hopkins Bayview Med Ctr, Baltimore, MD; Texas Tech Univ, Lubbock; Orthopaedic Surgery Specialists, Burbank, CA; et al)

J Hand Surg 37A:2636-2641, 2012

In growing numbers, patients are using social media platforms as resources to obtain health information and report their experiences in the health care setting. More physicians are making use of these platforms as a means to reach prospective and existing patients, to share information with each other, and to educate the public. In this ever-expanding online dialogue, questions have arisen regarding appropriate conduct of the physician during these interactions. The purpose of this article is to review the laws that govern online communication as they pertain to physician presence in this forum and to discuss appropriate ethical and professional behavior in this setting.

▶ Social media is here to stay. This article serves as a primer to review the laws governing online communication as they pertain to physician presence and to discuss appropriate ethical and professional behavior. Physicians must know the laws regarding the use of social media and take proactive steps to educate and protect themselves, their patients, and their practices. This is a must-read for anyone even peripherally involved with social media.

D. J. Smith, Jr, MD

Refinements in Pollicization: A 30-Year Experience
Taghinia AH, Littler JW, Upton J (St Luke's-Roosevelt Hosp, NY)
Plast Reconstr Surg 130:423e-433e, 2012

The thumb is a specialized organ with unique functions that cannot be replicated by any other digit. The most powerful technique for construction or reconstruction of a lost or missing thumb is index finger pollicization. In this article, the authors outline five technical refinements in this procedure that have evolved over the past 30 years in 313 cases. These refinements improve appearance and function, and include (1) modification of the incisions to produce a well-contoured web space, (2) metacarpal head positioning for optimal recreation of the carpal arch, (3) extrinsic tendon repositioning for improved pronation of the new thumb, (4) intrinsic tendon repositioning for maximal strength, and (5) thenar augmentation with an adipofascial flap in select cases for improved appearance.

▶ Pollicization is a powerful technique to construct/reconstruct a lost or missing thumb. The authors outline five technical refinements to improve appearance and function. They are (1) modification of the incisions to produce a well-contoured web space, (2) metacarpal head positioning for optimal recreation of the carpal arch, (3) extrinsic tendon repositioning for improved pronation of the new thumb, (4) intrinsic tendon repositioning for maximal strength, and (5) thenar augmentation with an adipofascial flap in select cases for improved appearance. With 30 years of experience and over more than 300 cases, this is a must-read for anyone doing this surgery.

D. J. Smith, Jr, MD

Toe-to-Hand Transfer: Evolving Indications and Relevant Outcomes
Waljee JF, Chung KC (Univ of Michigan Health System, Ann Arbor)
J Hand Surg 38A:1431-1434, 2013

Toe-to-hand transfer is indicated for many types of congenital and traumatic thumb absences. This review will highlight the applications of toe-to-hand transfer and their functional, aesthetic, and psychosocial outcomes. Despite its technical complexity, toe to hand reconstruction techniques can provide an elegant option to restore function for patients with difficult hand disabilities.

▶ Toe-to-hand transfer is indicated for many types of congenital and traumatic thumb absences. The authors emphasize the applications of toe-to-hand transfer and its functional, aesthetic, and psychosocial outcomes. This current concept is complete and concise. This is a nice review for those routinely performing the procedure and is a must-read for those who want to keep current.

D. J. Smith, Jr, MD

Inflammatory

Unraveling the signaling pathways promoting fibrosis in Dupuytren's disease reveals TNF as a therapeutic target

Verjee LS, Verhoekx JSN, Chan JKK, et al (Univ of Oxford, London, UK; et al)
Proc Natl Acad Sci U S A 110:E928-E937, 2013

Dupuytren's disease is a very common progressive fibrosis of the palm leading to flexion deformities of the digits that impair hand function. The cell responsible for development of the disease is the myofibroblast. There is currently no treatment for early disease or for preventing recurrence following surgical excision of affected tissue in advanced disease. Therefore, we sought to unravel the signaling pathways leading to the development of myofibroblasts in Dupuytren's disease. We characterized the cells present in Dupuytren's tissue and found significant numbers of immune cells, including classically activated macrophages. High levels of proinflammatory cytokines were also detected in tissue from Dupuytren's patients. We compared the effects of these cytokines on contraction and profibrotic signaling pathways in fibroblasts from the palmar and nonpalmar dermis of Dupuytren's patients and palmar fibroblasts from non-Dupuytren's patients. Exogenous addition of TNF, but not other cytokines, including IL-6 and IL-1β, promoted differentiation into specifically of palmar dermal fibroblasts from Dupuytren's patients in to myofibroblasts. We also demonstrated that TNF acts via the Wnt signaling pathway to drive contraction and profibrotic signaling in these cells. Finally, we examined the effects of targeted cytokine inhibition. Neutralizing antibodies to TNF inhibited the contractile activity of myofibroblasts derived from Dupuytren's patients, reduced their expression of α-smooth muscle actin, and mediated disassembly of the contractile apparatus. Therefore, we showed that localized inflammation in Dupuytren's disease contributes to the development and progression of this fibroproliferative disorder and identified TNF as a therapeutic target to down-regulate myofibroblast differentiation and activity.

► We are not often provided with an article to review from the *Proceedings of the National Academy of Sciences of the United States of America*. That is unfortunate. These authors note that the cell responsible for the progressive fibrosis in Dupuytren disease is the myofibroblast. They found that exogenous addition of only tumor necrosis factor (TNF) promoted differentiation of palmar dermal fibroblasts from Dupuytren patients into myofibroblasts. Conversely, neutralizing TNF inhibited the contractile ability. In summary, the authors showed that localized inflammation in Dupuytren disease contributes to the development and progression of this fibroproliferative disorder and identified TNF as a therapeutic target to downregulate myofibroblast differentiation and activity. A spectacular article! This is a well-presented, straightforward science and an excellent review for those who are scientifically inclined.

D. J. Smith, Jr, MD

Percutaneous Needle Fasciotomy for Recurrent Dupuytren Disease

van Rijssen AL, Werker PMN (Isala Clinics, Zwolle, The Netherlands)
J Hand Surg 37A:1820-1823, 2012

Purpose.—Increasing options to treat Dupuytren disease include percutaneous needle fasciotomy (PNF), a minimally invasive technique that has proven to be effective for the treatment of primary disease. However, its effect on recurrent disease is not clear.

Methods.—We studied 30 patients with recurrent Dupuytren disease in 40 fingers, with a mean follow-up of 4.4 years. Primary outcome measures were total passive extension deficit reduction and interval to a second recurrence, defined as an increase of more than 30° compared with the result at the end of the previous treatment. We noted complications.

Results.—Total passive extension reduction was 76%. Percutaneous needle fasciotomy was especially effective for the metacarpophalangeal joint, with an average reduction of 93%, whereas the average reduction in the proximal interphalangeal joint was 57%. A total of 50% of patients did not develop a secondary recurrence during follow-up. The other 50% did, and we treated recurrence within an average of 1.4 years after PNF. By means of PNF, we postponed tertiary treatment an average of 2.9 years starting from the initial treatment for Dupuytren disease. We successfully treated all secondary recurrences by limited fasciectomy, according to patients' wishes. We noted no major adverse effects.

Conclusions.—Percutaneous needle fasciotomy can be applied effectively for recurrent disease; 50% of patients remain free of recurrence for a mean of 4.4 years. If a secondary recurrence occurs, it does so relatively early after treatment. Patients must therefore be willing to accept this uncertainty in the context of the advantages of PNF, such as fast recovery, low complication rate, and minimal invasiveness.

Type of Study/Level of Evidence.—Therapeutic IV.

► Percutaneous needle fasciectomy (PNF) has proven effective in treating primary Dupuytren's disease. These authors began an evaluation of its effectiveness in recurrent disease. They found 50% without recurrence 4.4 years after treatment. Of the 50% that did recur, they recurred early, by an average of 1.4 years. PNF was more effective for metacarpophalangeal joint restriction. Assuming that larger numbers substantiate this observation, it seems a good alternative for the well-informed patient. Having 50% of patients not have a recurrence after 4.4 years with this minimally invasive procedure seems reasonable.

D. J. Smith, Jr, MD

Correction of Contracture and Recurrence Rates of Dupuytren Contracture Following Invasive Treatment: The Importance of Clear Definitions

Werker PMN, Pess GM, van Rijssen AL, et al (Univ of Groningen, the Netherlands; Central Jersey Hand Surgery, Eatontown, NJ; Drexel Univ School of Medicine, Philadelphia, PA; et al)

J Hand Surg 37A:2095-2105.e7, 2012

Purpose.—To call attention to the wide variety of definitions for recurrence that have been employed in studies of different invasive procedures for the treatment of Dupuytren contracture and how this important limitation has contributed to the wide range of reported results.

Methods.—This study reviewed definitions and rates of contracture correction and recurrence in patients undergoing invasive treatment of Dupuytren contracture. A literature search was carried out in January 2011 using the terms "Dupuytren" AND ("fasciectomy" OR "fasciotomy" OR "dermofasciectomy" OR "aponeurotomy" OR "aponeurectomy") and limited to studies in English.

Results.—The search returned 218 studies, of which 21 had definitions, quantitative results for contracture correction and recurrence, and a sample size of at least 20 patients. Definitions for correction of contracture and recurrence varied greatly among articles and were almost always qualitative. Percentages of patients who achieved correction of contracture (ie, responder rate) when evaluated at various times after completion of surgery ranged from 15% to 96% for fasciectomy/aponeurectomy. Responder rates were not reported for fasciotomy/aponeurotomy. Recurrence rates ranged from 12% to 73% for patients treated with fasciectomy/aponeurectomy and from 33% to 100% for fasciotomy/aponeurotomy. Review of these reports underscored the difficulty involved in comparing correction of contracture and recurrence rates for different surgical interventions because of differences in definition and duration of follow-up.

Conclusions.—Clearly defined objective definitions for correction of contracture and for recurrence are needed for more meaningful comparisons of results achieved with different surgical interventions.

Clinical Relevance.—Recurrence after surgical intervention for Dupuytren contracture is common. This study, which evaluated reported rates of recurrence following surgical treatment of Dupuytren contracture, provides clinicians with practical information regarding expected long-term outcomes of surgical treatment choices.

Type of Study/Level of Evidence.—Economic and decision analysis III.

▶ This study was designed to highlight the wide variety of definitions for recurrence that have been employed in studies of different invasive procedures for the treatment of Dupuytren's contracture and how this important limitation has contributed to the wide range of reported results. Definitions for correction of contracture and recurrence varied greatly and were almost always qualitative. This highlights the difficulty involved in comparing correction of contracture and recurrence rates for different surgical interventions because of differences in definition and duration of follow-up. As the importance of best practices increases, standardizing our evaluation tools is paramount. This article is important because it highlights the inadequacies that exist today. Hopefully, the next steps will involve attempts to standardize these definitions.

D. J. Smith, Jr, MD

The Effect of Night Extension Orthoses Following Surgical Release of Dupuytren Contracture: A Single-Center, Randomized, Controlled Trial

Collis J, Collocott S, Hing W, et al (Counties Manukau District Health Board, Auckland, New Zealand; AUT Univ, Auckland, New Zealand)

J Hand Surg 38:1285-1294.e2, 2013

Purpose.—To clarify the efficacy and detrimental effects of orthoses used to maintain finger extension following surgical release of Dupuytren contracture.

Methods.—We conducted a single-center, randomized, controlled trial to investigate the effect of night extension orthoses on finger range of motion and hand function for 3 months following surgical release of Dupuytren contracture. We also wanted to determine how well finger extension was maintained in the total sample. We randomized 56 patients to receive a night extension orthosis plus hand therapy (n = 26) or hand therapy alone (n = 30). The primary outcome was total active extension of the operated fingers (°). Secondary outcomes were total active flexion of the operated fingers (°), active distal palmar crease (cm), grip strength (kg), and self-reported hand function using the Disabilities of the Arm, Shoulder, and Hand questionnaire (0—100 scale).

Results.—There were no statistically significant differences between the no-orthosis and orthosis groups for total active extension or for any of the secondary outcomes. Between the first postoperative measure and 3 months after surgery, 62% of little fingers had maintained or improved total active extension.

Conclusions.—The use of a night extension orthosis in combination with standard hand therapy has no greater effect on maintaining finger extension than hand therapy alone in the 3 months following surgical release of Dupuytren contracture. Our results indicate that the practice of providing every patient with a night extension orthosis following surgical release of Dupuytren contracture may not be justified except for cases in which extension loss occurs after surgery. Our results also challenge clinicians to research ways of maintaining finger extension in a greater number of patients.

Type of Study/Level of Evidence.—Therapeutic II.

▶ The authors attempt to clarify the efficiency and detrimental effects of orthosis used to maintain finger extension after surgical release of Dupuytren contracture. They found the use of a night extension orthosis combined with standard hand therapy had no greater effect on maintaining finger extension than hand therapy alone in the 3 months after surgical release of Dupuytren contracture. Any time a study is able to challenge current trends it is worth evaluating. Even though there are deficiencies in the study (eg, single institution and power analysis), it is worth considering and possibly modifying postoperative care.

D. J. Smith, Jr, MD

Nerve

Endoscopic Carpal Tunnel Release Is Preferred Over Mini-open Despite Similar Outcome: A Randomized Trial

Kang HJ, Koh IH, Lee TJ, et al (Yonsei Univ College of Medicine, Seoul, Korea)
Clin Orthop Relat Res 471:1548-1554, 2013

Background.—The decision to perform endoscopic versus the mini-open carpal tunnel release technique is most likely left to surgeons rather than patients with idiopathic carpal tunnel syndrome.

Questions/Purposes.—We hypothesized that (1) at 3 months after surgery, the subjective outcomes of endoscopic release, performed on one hand, and mini-incision release, performed on the other, would not differ in patients with bilateral carpal tunnel syndrome; however, (2) each patient would likely prefer one technique over the other for specific reasons.

Methods.—Fifty-two patients with bilateral carpal tunnel syndrome had one hand randomized to undergo endoscopic release and the other to undergo mini-incision release. Each patient was assessed with the Boston Carpal Tunnel Questionnaire (BCTQ) and DASH preoperatively and at each followup. Three months after surgery, the patients commented on which technique they preferred and completed a questionnaire regarding the reasons for not preferring the other technique.

Results.—The mean BCTQ symptom/function score and DASH improved similarly in the endoscopic release group and the mini-incision release group. Thirty-four patients preferred endoscopic release and 13 preferred the mini-incision technique. Scar or pillar pain was the most commonly cited factor in not preferring either technique followed by postoperative pain for the open technique and transient worsening of symptoms for the endoscopic technique.

Conclusions.—Despite similar improvements in BCTQ and DASH scores after endoscopic and open techniques at 3 months postoperatively, the majority of our patients preferred the endoscopic technique. The most concerning reason for not preferring the other technique was scar or pillar pain.

▶ The authors randomly assigned patients with bilateral carpal tunnel syndrome to have one hand undergo endoscopic release and the other to undergo mini-incision release. Despite similar Boston Carpal Tunnel Questionnaire and Disabilities of the Arm, Shoulder and Hand scores after each procedure at 3 months postoperatively, most patients preferred the endoscopic technique. The most concerning reason for not preferring the other technique was scar or pillar pain. The number of patients is small. The discrimination is not great, but it is certainly an interesting trend. This is worth considering or at least engaging patients in your own practice.

D. J. Smith, Jr, MD

Trend of Recovery after Simple Decompression for Treatment of Ulnar Neuropathy at the Elbow

Giladi AM, For the Surgery of the Ulnar Nerve Study Group (Univ of Michigan Health System, Ann Arbor; et al)

Plast Reconstr Surg 131:563e-573e, 2013

Background.—Although numerous studies have investigated long-term outcomes after surgical treatment of ulnar neuropathy at the elbow with simple decompression, no study has evaluated the trend of postoperative recovery. The authors assessed timing of recovery after simple decompression for ulnar neuropathy at the elbow.

Methods.—The five-center Surgery of the Ulnar Nerve Study Group prospectively recruited 58 consecutive subjects with ulnar neuropathy at the elbow and treated them with simple decompression. Patients were evaluated preoperatively and at 6 weeks, 3 months, 6 months, and 1 year postoperatively. Patient-rated outcomes questionnaires included the Michigan Hand Questionnaire; the Disabilities of the Arm, Shoulder and Hand questionnaire; and the Carpal Tunnel Questionnaire. Functional tests used were grip strength, key pinch strength, two-point discrimination, and Semmes-Weinstein monofilament testing. Postoperative improvement was assessed at each time point to establish the trend of recovery in reaching a plateau.

Results.—Significant patient-reported symptomatic and functional recovery occurred over the first 6 weeks postoperatively as represented by improvements in questionnaire scores. Symptomatic recovery occurred earlier than functional recovery as measured by sensory and strength testing and the work domain of the Michigan Hand Questionnaire. Improvement in patient-reported outcomes continued and reached a plateau at 3 months, whereas measured strength and sensory recovery continued over 12 months.

Conclusion.—The greatest clinical improvement after simple decompression for ulnar neuropathy at the elbow, according to questionnaire scores, occurs in the first 6 weeks postoperatively and reaches a plateau by 3 months.

▶ The Surgery of the Ulnar Nerve Study Group is a collaboration of 5 centers. In this part of the study, the authors assessed timing of recovery after simple decompression for ulnar neuropathy at the elbow. They noted the greatest clinical improvement, according to questionnaire scores, occurs in the first 6 weeks postoperatively and reaches a plateau by 3 months. This group is working together effectively by pooling data. Even with that, the high percentage of patients (23%) lost has the potential to introduce attrition bias.

D. J. Smith, Jr, MD

The Minimal Clinically Important Difference After Simple Decompression for Ulnar Neuropathy at the Elbow

Malay S, SUN Study Group (Univ of Michigan Health System, Ann Arbor; et al)

J Hand Surg 38A:652-659, 2013

Purpose.—Establishing minimally clinically important difference (MCID) for patient-reported outcomes questionnaires is an important component of outcomes research to understand treatment effectiveness from the patient's perspective. For patients with ulnar neuropathy at the elbow (UNE), these assessments are vital to examine how much change in the questionnaire scores equate to patient satisfaction.

Methods.—We calculated the change in scores of Michigan Hand Outcomes Questionnaire (MHQ), Disabilities of the Arm, Shoulder, and Hand (DASH) questionnaire, and Carpal Tunnel Questionnaire (CTQ) from preoperative to 3, 6, and 12 months after ulnar nerve simple decompression procedure. We used the anchor-based approach of receiver operating characteristic curves to determine the MCID.

Results.—On average, MCID of 10, 12, and 7 points were identified for pain, function, and activities of daily living domains of the MHQ. Similarly, DASH, CTQ-symptom severity scale, and CTQ-function severity scale had an average MCID of 7, 0.7, and 0.3, points respectively. At the 3, 6, and 12 months' time points, an MCID of 9, 8, and 13 points for pain; 12, 12, and 12 points for function; and 6, 8, and 6 points for activities of daily living domains of the MHQ were identified; similarly an MCID of 8, 7, and 7 points for DASH; 0.4, 0.7, and 0.7 points for CTQ-symptom severity scale; and 0.3, 0.3, and 0.4 points for CTQ-function severity scale were established.

Conclusions.—The smaller MCIDs of MHQ, DASH, and even smaller MCIDs of CTQ found in our study indicate that a small change in the scores identified satisfied patients. Simple decompression surgery for UNE produced patient satisfaction with only a small change in their questionnaire scores. The implications of this finding are that simple decompression surgery for UNE is a highly effective procedure and that the outcomes questionnaires used are highly responsive, which minimizes sample size requirements for future research studies relating to UNE.

Type of Study/Level of Evidence.—Therapeutic II.

▶ Establishing minimally clinically important difference (MCID) for patient-reported outcomes questionnaires is an important component of outcomes research to understand treatment effectiveness from the patient's perspective. The MCID achieves several functions beyond serving as a measure for meaningful clinical improvement. First, MCID helps to estimate the required sample size so that a study has sufficient power to detect the true differences and, therefore, assess treatments better. Second, the ability to interpret study results accurately increases by understanding the implication of the change it scores. Despite several advantages, MCID has some limitations (eg, it is not a fixed value but varies with assessment methods). These authors determined that simple decompression of ulnar neuropathy at the elbow is a highly effective procedure and that the outcomes questionnaires used are highly responsive, which minimizes sample size requirements for future research studies relating to ulnar neuropathy at the elbow. This article is a must-read in this environment of evidence-based medicine.

D. J. Smith, Jr, MD

Functional Outcome Following Nerve Repair in the Upper Extremity Using Processed Nerve Allograft

Cho MS, Rinker BD, Weber RV, et al (Antonio Military Med Ctr, Fort Sam, Houston, TX; Univ of Kentucky, Lexington; Inst for Nerve, Hand, and Reconstructive Surgery, Rutherford, NJ; et al)

J Hand Surg 37A:2340-2349, 2012

Purpose.—Reconstruction of peripheral nerve discontinuities with processed nerve allograft has become increasingly relevant. The RANGER Study registry was initiated in 2007 to study the use of processed nerve allografts in contemporary clinical practice. We undertook this study to analyze outcomes for upper extremity nerve repairs contained in the registry database.

Methods.—We identified an upper extremity–specific population within the RANGER Study registry database consisting of 71 nerves repaired with processed nerve allograft. This group was composed of 56 subjects with a mean age of 40 ± 17 years (range, 18–86 y). We analyzed data to determine the safety and efficacy of processed nerve allograft. Quantitative data were available on 51 subjects with 35 sensory, 13 mixed, and 3 motor nerves. The mean gap length was 23 ± 12 mm (range, 5–50 mm). We performed an analysis to evaluate response-to-treatment and to examine sensory and motor recovery according to the international standards for motor and sensory nerve recovery.

Results.—There were no reported implant complications, tissue rejections, or adverse experiences related to the use of the processed nerve allografts. Overall recovery, S3 or M4 and above, was achieved in 86% of the procedures. Subgroup analysis demonstrated meaningful levels of recovery in sensory, mixed, and motor nerve repairs with graft lengths between 5 and 50 mm. The study also found meaningful levels of recovery in 89% of digital nerve repairs, 75% of median nerve repairs, and 67% of ulnar nerve repairs.

Conclusions.—Our data suggest that processed nerve allografts offer a safe and effective method of reconstructing peripheral nerve gaps from 5 to 50 mm in length. These outcomes compare favorably with those reported in the literature for nerve autograft, and exceed those reported for tube conduits.

Type of Study/Level of Evidence.—Therapeutic III.

▶ Nerve allografts provide organized microarchitecture, extracellular matrix constituents, and handling qualities of nerve autograft with the benefit and convenience of an off-the-shelf graft. Data are gradually being accumulated, and this report comes from the RANGER Study Registry Database. An upper extremity population identified 71 nerves repaired with processed nerve allograft. There were no implant complications, tissue rejections, or adverse experiences. The data show outcomes that compare favorably with those reported in the literature for nerve autograft—and exceed those reported for tube conduits. These are exciting results and show promise for the future. The availability of an off-the-shelf product with comparable results will simplify surgery and decrease time in the operating room.

D. J. Smith, Jr, MD

4 Aesthetic

Face, Neck, and Brow

Hair Restoration Surgery: The State of the Art

Vogel JE, Jimenez F, Cole J, et al (The Johns Hopkins Hosp and School of Medicine, Baltimore, MD; Private Practice in Canary Islands, Spain; Private Practice in Alpharetta, GA; et al)

Aesthet Surg J 33:128-151, 2013

Hair restoration is a highly sophisticated subspecialty that offers significant relief to patients with hair loss. An improved understanding of the aesthetics of hair loss and cosmetic hair restoration, hair anatomy and physiology, and the development of microvascular surgical instrumentation has revolutionized the approach to surgical hair restoration since the original description. Additional elements that contribute to the current state of the art in hair restoration include graft size, site creation, packing density, and medical control of hair loss. The results of hair restoration are natural in appearance and are provided with a very high level of patient satisfaction and safety. This aspect of cosmetic surgery is a very welcome addition to a traditional aesthetic practice and serves as a tremendous source for internal cross-referral. The future of hair restoration surgery is centered on minimal-incision surgery as well as cell-based therapies.

▶ Hair restoration procedures continue to be in demand as procedural techniques yield more natural results. The introduction of automated follicular unit extraction devices and, more recently, robotic technology has drawn more patient interest. This review offers an update on recent advances in the field by experienced hair restoration specialists.

K. A. Gutowski, MD

Fractional CO_2 Laser Treatment vs Autologous Fat Transfer in the Treatment of Acne Scars: A Comparative Study

Azzam OA, Atta AT, Sobhi RM, et al (Cairo Univ, Egypt)
J Drugs Dermatol 12:e7-e13, 2013

Background.—Acne scars present a highly challenging and frustrating clinical problem. Fractional CO_2 laser treatment has led to marked improvement in scars, and fat transfer, or fat grafting, has also recently proven very useful in regenerative medicine.

Objective.—To compare fractional CO_2 laser treatment and fat grafting in the treatment of acne scars.

Materials and Methods.—Twenty patients were included in this study, 10 received 3 sessions of fractional CO_2 laser therapy, and 10 received fat grafting. All patients were then followed up for 3 months, and results were assessed with digital photographs taken by a committee of 3 physicians, by a single-blinded physician, and by reports of patient satisfaction.

Results.—In the fractional CO_2 laser treatment group, under 20% of patients were graded as having excellent scar improvement, 0 as having marked scar improvement, under 10% as having mild scar improvement, and almost 70% as having moderate scar improvement. In the fat-grafting group, the scar and overall improvement were graded as 30% excellent, 30% marked, 20% moderate, and 20% mild.

Conclusion.—Fat grafting proved to be more effective in the treatment of acne scars than ablative fractional CO_2 laser treatment. There were many points in its favor, the most significant being the clinical improvement in scars and texture. This supports the stem cell theory of adipose tissue in regenerative medicine.

▶ Others have also reported favorable results with fat transfer when treating acne scars. The 3-month endpoint in this study may be too short for a true comparison, as the effects of both CO_2 lasers and fat transfer may evolve for 6 months or more. Because there are different types of acne scars, it is important to match the treatment to the type of scar. In this study, patients with ice pick scars showed no improvement from fat transfer (and they typically do not improve with ablative laser treatment). Perhaps future studies will evaluate combination treatment with laser and fat transfer.

K. A. Gutowski, MD

Comparison of a Fractional Microplasma Radio Frequency Technology and Carbon Dioxide Fractional Laser for the Treatment of Atrophic Acne Scars: A Randomized Split-Face Clinical Study

Zhang Z, Fei Y, Chen X, et al (Shanghai JiaoTong Univ, China)
Dermatol Surg 39:559-566, 2013

Background.—No studies have compared fractional microplasma radio frequency (RF) technology with the carbon dioxide fractional laser system (CO_2 FS) in the treatment of atrophic acne scars in the same patient.

Objective.—To compare the efficacy and safety of fractional microplasma RF with CO_2 FS in the treatment of atrophic acne scars.

Methods and Materials.—Thirty-three Asian patients received three sessions of a randomized split-face treatment of fractional microplasma RF or CO_2 FS.

Results.—Both modalities had a roughly equivalent effect. Échelle d'Évaluation Clinique Des Cicatrices d'Acné scores were significantly lower after fractional microplasma RF (from 51.1 ± 14.2 to 22.3 ± 8.6, 56.4% improvement) and CO_2 FS (from 48.8 ± 15.1 to 19.9 ± 7.9, 59.2% improvement) treatments. There was no statistically significant difference between the two therapies. Twelve subjects (36.4%) experienced postinflammatory hyperpigmentation (PIH) after 30 of 99 treatment sessions (30.3%) on the CO_2 FS side and no PIH was observed on the fractional microplasma RF sides.

Conclusion.—Both modalities have good effects on treating atrophic scars. PIH was not seen with the fractional microplasma RF, which might make it a better choice for patients with darker skin.

▶ CO_2 lasers work well for improving acne scars but have limitations in patients with skin types Fitzpatrick III and higher caused by hyperpigmentation. Radiofrequency is a newer technology that delivers thermal energy to deeper tissue and can be used in a fractional mode. This study suggests that fractional radiofrequency modalities may be useful in treating patients who have darker skin types without the risks of postinflammatory hyperpigmentation.

K. A. Gutowski, MD

Augmentation of the Upper Lip With Temporalis Fascia: A Quantitative Analysis

Bohluli B, Amirzargar R, Moharamnejad N (Buali Hosp, Tehran, Iran; Azad Univ of Med Sciences, Tehran, Iran; Shariati Hosp, Tehran, Iran)
Aesthet Surg J 33:102-108, 2013

Background.—Lip augmentation is a very common cosmetic procedure. A wide variety of materials have been used to enhance and contour the lips, including alloplastic and autogenous substances.

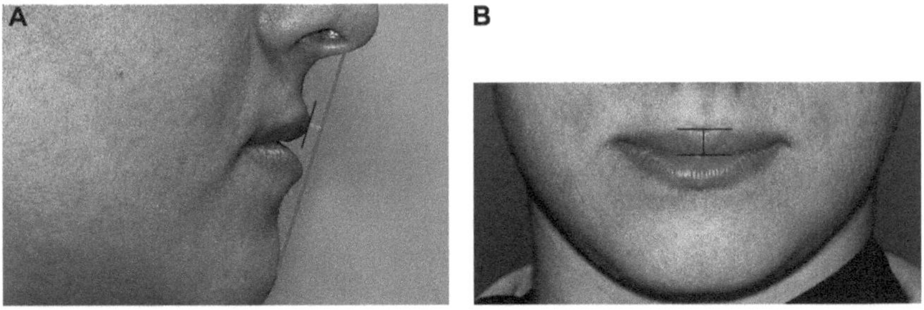

FIGURE 3.—(A) Measurement of upper-lip projection. Steiner's line is indicated in red. The value of the projection is indicated in green. (B) Measurement of upper-lip vermilion show. (Reprinted from Bohluli B, Amirzargar R, Moharamnejad N. Augmentation of the upper lip with temporalis fascia: a quantitative analysis. *Aesthet Surg J*. 2013;33:102-108, © 2013, Aesthetic Surgery Journal.)

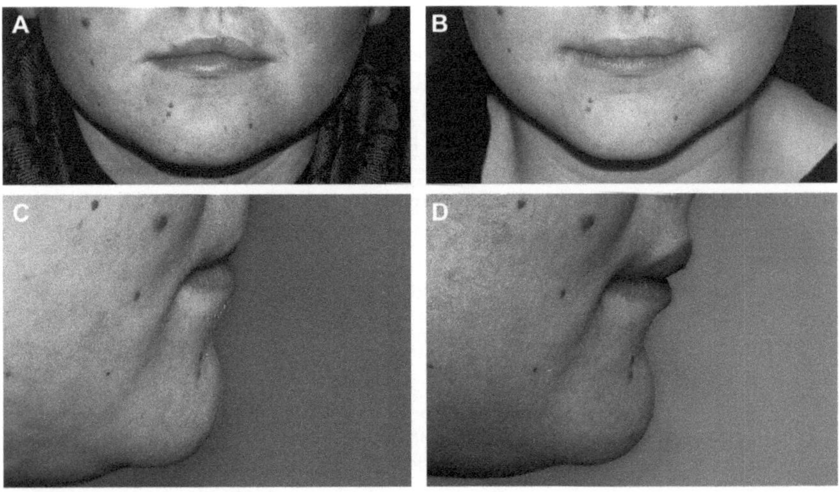

FIGURE 4.—(A, C) This 20-year-old woman presented with a cleft lip. (B, D) Six months after augmentation of the upper lip with temporalis fascia. (Reprinted from Bohluli B, Amirzargar R, Moharamnejad N. Augmentation of the upper lip with temporalis fascia: a quantitative analysis. *Aesthet Surg J*. 2013;33:102-108, © 2013, Aesthetic Surgery Journal.)

Objectives.—The authors describe their experience with augmentation of the upper lip using an autologous graft from the temporalis fascia.

Methods.—Patients were enrolled prospectively. Upper-lip projection and vermilion show were measured preoperatively and 6 months postoperatively for 19 patients who were candidates for lip augmentation with temporalis fascia.

Results.—Six months postoperatively, the mean values for upper-lip projection and lip vermilion were significantly greater than preoperative measurements.

Conclusions.—Augmentation of the upper lip with temporalis fascia appears to be safe and effective. Larger patient series, longer follow-up, and comparative studies are needed to corroborate these preliminary results (Figs 3 and 4).

▶ Temporalis fascia is an extremely useful filling material for smaller facial defects, especially those involving the lips. I have used this material in a wide variety of cases and found it to be excellent. These authors' statistical analysis provides evidence of the efficacy of the technique, although most of the photos in the original article show only slight improvement. Some of the best improvements are in patients with cleft lip (Figs 3 and 4). I believe that better results might have occurred if the grafts were larger in volume, easily accomplished using the temporalis fascia without causing donor site deformity. In addition to placement of the fascia as described, I have placed the fascia into tunnels after opening the cleft lip scar in preparation for its revision.

S. H. Miller, MD

Excessive gingival display: Treatment by a modified lip repositioning technique

Silva CO, Ribeiro-Júnior NV, Campos TVS, et al (State Univ of Maringá (UEM)/Ingá Univ (UNINGÁ) Paraná, Maringá, Brazil; Alfenas Federal Univ (Unifal-MG), Minas Gerais, Brazil; et al)

J Clin Periodontol 40:260-265, 2013

Aim.—The objective of this prospective study was to investigate outcomes of a lip repositioning technique for the treatment of excessive gingival display.

Materials and Methods.—Thirteen consecutively treated patients with excessive gingival display were treated with a modified lip repositioning technique. Treatment consisted of the removal of two strips of mucosa, bilaterally to the maxillary labial frenum and coronal repositioning of the new mucosal margin. The clinical dimensions of gingival display, upper lip and vermillion length were measured at baseline, 3 and 6 months postoperatively. Subjects completed surveys to evaluate satisfaction with outcomes.

Results.—The baseline gingival display of 5.8 ± 2.1 mm significantly decreased to 1.4 ± 1.0 mm at 3 months ($p < 0.0001$) and was maintained until 6 months (1.3 ± 1.6 mm). The reduction in gingival display strongly correlated to the combined change in upper lip and vermillion length ($r^2 = 0.60$, $p = 0.0018$). Subjects were satisfied with their smile after surgery and would likely choose to undergo the procedure again (92%). The worst part of undergoing the procedure was the discomfort or the inability to move the lip during the early healing (69%).

Conclusion.—Treatment of excessive gingival display by means of a modified lip repositioning technique results in high level of patient satisfaction and predictable outcomes that are stable in the short term.

▶ The gummy smile caused by excessive upper gingival display may be caused by a vertical maxillary excess, anterior dentoalveolar extrusion, altered passive eruption (downward gingival migration), short or hyperactive upper lip, or a combination of these findings. If the upper lip length is normal and the lower facial third is not disproportionate, a hyperactive upper lip is considered the main cause of a gummy smile. In such cases, treatments include botulinum toxin, lip elongation associated with rhinoplasty, detachment of lip muscles, myotomy and partial removal, and lip repositioning. The lip repositioning procedure has been described by other authors in small patient series, and in most cases it seems to yield good results. Although it may be more commonly discussed among oral surgeons and dental surgeons, plastic surgeons should be aware of this simple treatment for a gummy smile.

K. A. Gutowski, MD

Exploratory, Randomized, Controlled, Phase 2 Study to Evaluate the Safety and Efficacy of Adjuvant Fibrin Sealant VH S/D 4 S-Apr (ARTISS) in Patients Undergoing Rhytidectomy

Hester TR Jr, Gerut ZE, Shire JR, et al (Private Practice in Atlanta, GA; Private Practice in Hewlett, NY; Private Practice in Chattanooga, TN; et al)
Aesthet Surg J 33:323-333, 2013

Background.—Suction drains are commonly placed after rhytidectomy surgery to avoid seroma formation that may result from dead spaces between skin layers. Fibrin sealants promote tissue adherence by cross-linking with extracellular matrix proteins, which may reduce the dead space under skin flaps.

Objectives.—The authors evaluate the safety and preliminary efficacy of the fibrin sealant (FS) VH S/D 4 s-apr (ARTISS; Baxter Healthcare Corp, Deerfield, Illinois), added to standard-of-care (SoC) treatment, on tissue plane adherence and local hemostasis in rhytidectomy patients.

Methods.—In this phase 2, prospective, controlled, randomized, evaluator- and patient-blinded, multicenter study, 45 patients (of 56 possible enrollees) received SoC treatment on 1 side of the face and adjunctive FS VH S/D 4 s-apr treatment on the other side. Outcomes measures included visual assessments of ecchymosis (by blinded reviewers), grading of ecchymosis and edema, drainage volumes, occurrence of hematoma/seroma, safety evaluations, and patient-reported assessments of pain, numbness, and treatment preferences postoperatively.

Results.—Mean patient age was 55.1 years. Rates and grades of ecchymosis and edema were similar for the 2 treatments. The mean (SD) drainage volume 24 hours after surgery was 11.5 (13.7) mL from the FS VH S/D 4 s-apr-treated sides of the face and 26.8 (24.0) mL from the

SoC-only sides ($P < .0001$). Patient assessments of pain, numbness, and preference favored treatment with FS VH S/D 4 s-apr. Adverse events were mild to moderate in severity.

Conclusions.—Adjuvant use of FS VH S/D 4 s-apr appears to be safe and results in lower drainage volumes than SoC treatment alone.

▶ Tissue sealants in aesthetic surgery have been promoted to reduce edema, ecchymosis, hematoma and seroma formation, and the need for drains. Reports vary on their usefulness in facelifts, and their use results in increased costs without consistently improved results.

In this study, the fibrin tissue sealant product did show statistically significant improvement in clinical endpoints. However, although the reduction in drain output from 14 mL to 24 mL over 24 hours may be statistically significant, it may not be clinically significant. Furthermore, blinded reviewers most commonly found that there was equal ecchymosis between the 2 groups (as opposed to a difference in ecchymosis between the groups) at postoperative days 1, 5, 7, 10, and 14, although on day 3 more subjects had less ecchymosis in the nonsealant group than in the sealant group. Hematoma and seroma rates were lower in the fibrin tissue sealant group, however. Based on this exploratory study, there does not seem to be an advantage in using this product to reduce ecchymosis, but it may decrease hematoma formation.

K. A. Gutowski, MD

Antidepressants and Bleeding Risk After Face-Lift Surgery

Harirchian S, Zoumalan RA, Rosenberg DB (Univ of Medicine and Dentistry of New Jersey, Newark; Facial Plastic and Reconstructive Surgery (private practice), Beverly Hills, CA; Manhattan Eye, Ear, and Throat Hospital, New York)
Arch Facial Plast Surg 14:248-252, 2012

Objective.—To determine the rate of post–face-lift hematoma among users of serotonin reuptake inhibitors (SSRIs) vs non-SSRI users. Selective serotonin reuptake inhibitors have come under recent scrutiny because of possible bleeding risks. However, cessation of SSRIs carries inherent risks.

Methods.—The medical charts for 250 consecutive patients who underwent a modified deep-plane face-lift and 13 patients who underwent neck-lift from January 2010 to May 2011 were reviewed for the incidence of postoperative hematoma. Patients' medical records were examined for medical comorbidities, coagulopathy, and medication list, with particular attention to any usage of SSRIs or serotonin norepinephrine reuptake inhibitors (SNRIs).

Results.—Twenty-two percent of patients were taking SSRIs or SNRIs. We observed a total hematoma (major + minor) rate of 1.95% for non–SSRI/SNRI users vs 1.72% for SSRI/SNRI users. The minor hematoma rate was 1.95%among nonusers vs 0% for users. The major hematoma rate was 0% among nonusers vs 1.72% for users.

Conclusions.—Usage of SSRIs was more common in this large series of face-lift patients than in the general population. In these patients, SSRIs in the perioperative period are found to be safe and did not seem to adversely affect outcome. We found no evidence to support discontinuing SSRIs perioperatively.

► Serotonin reuptake inhibitor (SSRI) antidepressants were found to increase the risk for reoperation because of bleeding in mastectomy patients and to increase intraoperative blood loss in hip arthroplasty patients. The increased bleeding may be due to SSRI inhibition of platelet aggregation. Although plastic surgeons typically ask their patients to stop all medications that may increase the risk of bleeding, discontinuing SSRI may increase the risk of psychological, gastrointestinal, and neurological complaints, including withdrawal symptoms. More serious symptoms included relapses in significant depression, aggression, hypomania, and suicide after discontinuing antidepressants. Discontinuation symptoms have been reported in 12% to 50% of antidepressant users beginning within 3 to 5 days of treatment cessation, and lasting up to 3 weeks. Although this study patient sample size did not have enough power to detect a small increase in bleeding risk, it does suggest that continuing SSRI medications during facial procedures does not adversely affect bleeding.

K. A. Gutowski, MD

Preauricular Incision Outlining During a Face-Lift: A Step-by-Step Description

Albertal JM, Davalos G, Leonetti M, et al (Tornu Hosp, Buenos Aires, Argentina; Private Practice, Buenos Aires, Argentina; et al)

Aesthetic Plast Surg 36:857-861, 2012

The data on the proper way to establish the preauricular incision (PAI) line and manage skin tension during lifting are limited. Undoubtedly, proper tissue handling represents a true challenge during a lifting procedure and is a crucial step in avoiding disfiguration. The authors describe their approach to PAI demarcation and local skin tension management performed in 165 cases since 2007.

Level of Evidence V.—This journal requires that authors assign a level of evidence to each article. For a full description of these Evidence-Based Medicine ratings, please refer to the Table of Contents or the online Instructions to Authors at www.springer.com/00266.

► Sometimes it is worthwhile to go back to the basics and focus on the fine details of surgical technique to improve results. This report gives useful step-by-step directions for designing a preauricular incision that leaves a natural result without the typical signs of a facelift (ie, wide scars, tragal distortion, pixie ear deformity). It is worthwhile to review and implement the recommendations.

K. A. Gutowski, MD

Patient-Specific Rhytidectomy: Finding the Angle of Maximal Rejuvenation

Jacono AA, Ransom ER (North Shore Univ Hosp, Manhasset, NY; Albert Einstein College of Medicine, Bronx, NY)

Aesthet Surg J 32:804-813, 2012

Background.—Rhytidectomy is fundamentally an operation of tissue release and resuspension, although the manner and direction of suspension are subject to perpetual debate.

Objectives.—The authors describe a method for identifying the angle of maximal rejuvenation during rhytidectomy and quantify the resulting angle and its relationship to patient age.

Methods.—Patients were prospectively enrolled; demographic data, history, and operative details were recorded. Rhytidectomies were performed by the senior author (AAJ). After complete elevation, the face-lift flap was rotated in a medially-based arc (0-90°) while attention was given to the submental area, jawline, and midface. The angle of maximal rejuvenation for each hemiface was identified as described, and the flap was resuspended. During redraping, measurements of vertical and horizontal skin excess were recorded in situ. The resulting angle of lift was then calculated for each hemiface using trigonometry. Symmetry between sides was determined, and the effect of patient age on this angle was assessed.

Results.—Three hundred hemifaces were operated (147 women; 3 men). Mean age was 60 years (range, 37-80 years). Mean resulting angle for the cohort was 60° from horizontal (range, 46-77°). This was inversely correlated with patient age ($r = -0.3$). Younger patients (<50 years, 64°) had a significantly more vertical angle than older patients (≥70 years, 56°; $P < .0002$). No significant intersubject difference was found between hemifaces ($P = .53$).

Conclusions.—The authors present a method for identifying the angle of maximal rejuvenation during rhytidectomy. This angle was more superior than posterior in all cases and is intimately related to patient age. Lasting results demand a detailed anatomical understanding and strict attention to the direction and degree of laxity.

► This article describes the effects of different facelift flap orientation angles on facial anatomic regions. Pulling in an overly horizontal direction results in tightening of the flap directly against the hyoid and infrahyoid neck, leaving the submental area relatively loose and causing bunching or residual redundancy. It also flattens the midface and tightens the skin over the infraorbital rim, accentuating the hollow in this area and contributing to the "wind-swept" look. Pulling in an overly vertical direction results in tightening of the flap directly against the suprahyoid neck and mandible, leaving residual laxity in the anterior neck. It also causes midfacial bunching in the lateral canthal region and may lead to vertical pleats in the lateral neck and changes in apparent eye shape from tissue excess at the lateral canthus.

By using a patient-specific angle of maximal rejuvenation (about 60 degrees), the deep tissues of the face and neck, along with the overlying skin, are tightened into the concavity of the cervicomental angle along the hyoid attachments. The midfacial tissues are also repositioned, resulting in revolumization and rejuvenation of the malar-infraorbital complex. Although the authors performed a deep plane facelift in all patients, the principles may be applied to a variety of facelift techniques (superficial musculoaponeurotic system [SMAS] plication, SMAS-ectomy, minimal access cranial suspension lift). This is different from some traditional teaching, where the SMAS is lifted vertically but the skin is redraped mostly horizontally.

K. A. Gutowski, MD

Anatomic Study of the Retaining Ligaments of the Face and Applications for Facial Rejuvenation

Rossell-Perry P, Paredes-Leandro P (Jockey Salud Med Ctr, Miraflores, Lima, Peru)

Aesthetic Plast Surg 37:504-512, 2013

Background.—The retaining ligaments of the face support the facial soft tissue in a normal anatomic position, thereby resisting gravitational change. In this study, a technique utilizing surgical plication of the superficial musculoaponeurotic system (SMAS) to the retaining ligaments of the face and finger-assisted malar elevation (FAME) dissection of the midface is presented.

Methods.—The anatomy of the facial retaining ligaments was studied in 20 half-faces of ten fresh cadavers, and the localization of the ligaments was examined macroscopically. Surgical correction of facial aging with plication of the SMAS to the retaining ligaments and FAME dissection of the midface has been performed in 74 face-lift patients since 2006. Outcomes were determined by case notes, clinical review, and a patient questionnaire.

Results.—The studied ligaments (zygomatic and masseteric) were present in all cadaver dissections. The zygomatic ligament was located 4.3–5.5 cm from the tragus and originates near the inferior border of the anterior zygomatic arch. The masseteric ligament was located 3.7–5.2 cm from the tragus below the junction of the zygomatic arch and masseter muscle. All the patients answered a satisfaction questionnaire and reported high levels of satisfaction at least 1 year after treatment.

Conclusions.—We have identified the facial retaining ligaments in all cadaver dissections and their relationship with other structures of the face are described here. This study demonstrates that our face-lift technique is safe and produces highly predictable and natural results.

Level of Evidence IV.—This journal requires that authors assign a level of evidence to each article. For a full description of these Evidence-Based

Medicine ratings, please refer to the Table of Contents or the online Instructions to Authors www.springer.com/00266.

▶ It is worthwhile to review the anatomy of the retaining ligaments and understand their importance in proper facelift dissection. However, based on the visual results, it is difficult to judge if the technique presented in this article is any better than a conventional superficial musculoaponeurotic system procedure.

K. A. Gutowski, MD

Anatomical Landmarks to Avoid Injury to the Great Auricular Nerve During Rhytidectomy

Lefkowitz T, Hazani R, Chowdhry S, et al (Manhattan Eye, Ear, and Throat Hosp/Lenox Hill Hosp, NY; Harvard Med School, Boston, MA; Univ of Louisville School of Medicine, KY)

Aesthet Surg J 33:19-23, 2013

Background.—An estimated 116 086 facelifts were performed in 2011. Regardless of the technique employed, facial flap elevation carries with it anatomical pitfalls of which any surgeon performing these procedures should be aware. Injury to the great auricular nerve (GAN) is the most common of these injuries, occurring at a rate of 6% to 7%.

Objectives.—We report our findings on the location of the GAN on the basis of anatomical landmarks to aid surgeons with planning their surgical approach for safe elevation of rhytidectomy skin flaps in the lateral neck region.

Methods.—Sixteen fresh cadaveric heads were dissected under loupe magnification. All specimens were dissected in a 45-degree (facelift) position in which a mid-sternocleidomastoid (SCM) incision was used for exposure. Measurements from the bony mastoid process, bony external auditory canal, external jugular vein, and anterior border of the SCM to the GAN were taken in each cadaver.

Results.—The GAN follows a consistent course over the mid-body of the SCM before bifurcating into anterior and posterior branches and terminal arborization. Regardless of the length of the SCM, the GAN at its most superficial location was found to be consistently at a ratio of one-third the distance from either the mastoid process or the external auditory canal to the clavicular origin of the SCM.

Conclusions.—Knowledge of the anatomy, course, and location of the GAN along the surface of SCM muscle based on anatomic landmarks and distance ratios can facilitate a safer dissection in the lateral neck during rhytidectomy procedures.

▶ Previous work by McKinney and others reported that the great auricular nerve (GAN) crosses the sternocleidomastoid muscle at about 6.5 cm inferior to the external auditory canal. This report suggests that taking a patient's body habitus into account, a ratio of anatomic distances, rather than absolute measurements, may be better at predicting the GAN location.

K. A. Gutowski, MD

Facelift Complications and the Risk of Venous Thromboembolism: A Single Center's Experience

Abboushi N, Yezhelyev M, Symbas J, et al (Plastic surgeons in private practice, Atlanta, GA; Emory Univ, Atlanta, GA)

Aesthet Surg J 32:413-420, 2012

Background.—The number of facelifts performed in the United States has steadily increased over the past decade. Moreover, the risk of venous thromboembolism in plastic surgery has been established in recent studies.

Objectives.—The authors investigate the overall complication rate in a single-center series to identify risk factors and determine the risk of venous thromboembolism.

Methods.—A retrospective chart review was performed for patients who underwent a facelift procedure at a private clinic in Atlanta, Georgia, between January 2004 and December 2010. A total of 630 patients were included. The data collected included patient demographics, comorbidities, body mass index, smoking history, operative time, and concurrent procedures. All postoperative complications were recorded.

Results.—The mean age of the patients in this series was 58.4 ± 7.3 years. A small percentage of the patients were men (8.1%); 23.2% had hypertension; 4.9% were smokers; and 3.5% had a history of taking prophylactic aspirin. The mean operative time was 255.6 ± 81.6 minutes. Almost a quarter (23.6%) of the patients underwent concurrent procedures. There were 38 complications, including 29 hematomas, two deep vein thromboses (DVTs), two eye infections, two instances of partial skin loss, and one ectropion. Risk of complications was significantly higher in men, patients over 55, and those with a body mass index >30 kg/m^2. The risk of hematoma was higher ($P < .05$) in men, patients over 55, those with a history of hypertension, and those taking aspirin. The risk of DVT increased when the procedure time was longer than five hours. Both patients who developed DVT had undergone a facelift in combination with another procedure. There was also an increase in the risk of complications when the facelift was combined with two or more procedures.

Conclusions.—Identifying various risk factors for complications, especially DVT, can help to minimize those factors in the postoperative period and treat complications effectively when they occur. The data indicate that the number of concurrent procedures is a specific risk factor for development of DVT, so care should be taken when planning for multiple treatment sites. Combining facelift with other procedures also increases the risk of complications, especially DVT.

Level of Evidence.—4.

▶ This study adds further support to proceeding with caution when planning multiprocedure operations that exceed 5 to 6 hours. There seems to be a higher risk of deep vein thrombosis (DVT) and pulmonary embolism (PE) in such cases, and, therefore, proper screening and DVT prophylaxis must be done. Consideration should be given to staging procedures when possible. Unfortunately, this study did not report the type of anesthesia used for these procedures. Other series have shown lower DVT and PE rates with monitored anesthesia care vs general anesthesia.

K. A. Gutowski, MD

The Staged Face Lift: Addressing the Biomechanical Limitations of the Primary Rhytidectomy

Rawlani V, Mustoe TA (Northwestern Univ, Chicago, IL)
Plast Reconstr Surg 130:1305-1314, 2012

Background.—Although early secondary face lift is a highly scrutinized procedure, it is beneficial for a select group of patients. Justification for performing the early secondary face lift or staged face lift is more apparent when considering the biomechanical limitations of the primary face lift.

Methods.—All patients undergoing primary face-lift procedures performed by the senior author (T.A.M.) between 1998 and 2008 were followed for 2 years to determine which patients would benefit from an early secondary rhytidectomy. Early secondary face lifts were performed in the same sub–superficial musculoaponeurotic system plane as the primary procedure and entailed full undermining.

Results.—Forty-seven of 742 patients (6.3 percent) undergoing a primary face-lift procedure underwent an early secondary rhytidectomy. Identified limiting factors of the primary face lift included suture-tearing force, viscoelastic properties (tissue creep and stress relaxation), blood supply, and an attempt to avoid an overly pulled appearance. Indications for early secondary rhytidectomy included early symptoms of recurrence or residual age-related changes in patients with severe preoperative laxity or poor soft-tissue elasticity and mainly involved the perioral region. There were no significant complications and there was high patient satisfaction in all cases.

Conclusion.—With thorough understanding of the viscoelastic properties of facial tissues and proper consultation with patients, the early secondary face lift can be used as a safe and effective option with which to address the limitations of a primary face lift.

Clinical Question/Level of Evidence.—Therapeutic, IV.

▶ Most facelift surgeons have patients whose results do not meet their own, and their patient's, expectations. As hard as it may be to suggest a second facelift within 1 to 2 years, if the patient is approached properly, significant improvement can be achieved. As the authors point out, the key to successfully incorporating the early secondary rhytidectomy into one's practice is appropriate consultation. Unless this is made emphatically clear at the outset, there will be patients who think that the results of a single facelift operation will completely rejuvenate their face and neck and last indefinitely. Although it is difficult to fully predict who will require a secondary procedure, one should generally expect a 20% recurrence of symptoms. In patients with severe laxity and poor elasticity—specifically, in the perioral or central neck region—an 80% correction may not be sufficient to meet the expectations of the patient, and a secondary procedure may be anticipated.

K. A. Gutowski, MD

How Long Does a Face Lift Last? Objective and Subjective Measurements over a 5-Year Period

Jones BM, Lo SJ (King Edward VII's Sister Agnes Hosp, London, Glasgow, UK)

Plast Reconstr Surg 130:1317-1327, 2012

Background.—The longevity of face-lift surgery is a key question that has not been adequately addressed by previous studies. No study has used standardized photographs, objective measurements, or validated subjective scoring systems.

Methods.—From 2001 to 2011, photographs were standardized in this institution. Fifty primary face-lift patients were assessed 5.5 years after surgery using objective measurements from standardized photographs, a region-specific subjective assessment (Scale Summit II scores), and an overall subjective assessment (Global Aesthetic Improvement Scores).

Results.—For the first outcome measure, the jowl elevated in vertical height by 6 mm after face-lift surgery, with a relapse of 21 percent at 5.5 years. Jowl correction was maintained at 5.5-year follow-up ($p < 0.0001$). Cervicomental angle decreased by 13 degrees after face-lift surgery, with partial relapse of 69 percent at 5.5 years. For the second outcome measure, scores showed significant improvement in all areas following a face lift (jowl, nasolabial, and marionette, $p < 0.0001$; neck, $p = 0.0007$). At 5.5 years, no subjective worsening of any area was noted except the neck. For the third outcome measure, scoring suggested that 76 percent of patients will still appear younger 5.5 years after a face lift than they did before the face lift.

Conclusions.—This study indicates that differential regional aging occurs after face lifting, with the jowl, nasolabial, and marionette areas remaining well corrected at 5.5 years but with partial relapse of neck correction. Long-term global aesthetic assessment remains positive in the vast majority of patients. This study provides strong evidence that face-lift surgery can provide significant long-term aesthetic gains.

Clinical Question/Level of Evidence.—Therapeutic, IV.

► A common question asked by patients considering a facelift is, "how long will it last?" Most surgeons feel that the best answer is something related to "resetting of the aging clock" and that the normal aging process will continue. Based on a limited number of studies, a facelift may make a patient appear about 10 years younger, and patients seem to have secondary facelifts about 10 years or later after the first procedure. Some studies have found longer lasting results with more extensive techniques, but given the difficulty of measuring long-term outcomes, there is no consensus on which technique really lasts longer.

This study used standardized and objective measurements to show that improvements are maintained most efficiently in the jowl and marionette regions but to a lesser degree in the neck, suggesting that there is a regional vs a global facial aging process. Patients may be advised of the different ranges of facelift duration and that the neck may age faster than the face.

K. A. Gutowski, MD

A 20-Year Experience with Secondary Rhytidectomy: A Review of Technique, Longevity, and Outcomes

Beale EW, Rasko Y, Rohrich RJ (Univ of Texas Southwestern Med Ctr, Dallas)
Plast Reconstr Surg 131:625-634, 2013

Background.—The increasingly more common secondary rhytidectomy patient presents with recurrent soft-tissue descent and stigmata of primary face lift, which can require techniques unique to secondary rhytidectomy. The senior author's (R.J.R.) experience with secondary rhytidectomy is reviewed, focusing on surgical technique, longevity, and outcomes.

Methods.—Data collected after chart review of a 20-year study period included face-lift technique; duration between primary, secondary, and tertiary face lifts; concurrent procedures; and complications (i.e., hematoma, seroma, nerve injury, skin slough, infection, and need for revision). Surgical technique focuses on the "five Rs" of secondary rhytidectomy: (1) resect skin/scar, (2) release of abnormal superficial musculoaponeurotic system (SMAS) vectors, (3) refill by means of fat grafting, (4) reshape with SMASectomy or SMAS-stacking plication, and (5) redrape skin. The longevity of primary and secondary procedures was compared.

Results.—A total of 811 face lifts were performed during the study period; 60 were secondary procedures. Ten secondary patients went on to have a tertiary face lift. Average duration between primary and secondary face lift was 9.0 years, and that between secondary and tertiary procedures was 7.5 years, showing no difference in longevity ($p = 0.2$). Complications included one each of seroma, skin slough, and temporary marginal mandibular nerve injury (2 percent). Necessary revisions included one neck, one earlobe, and one preauricular scar.

Conclusions.—Secondary rhytidectomy has complications similar to those of a primary procedure, and most patients have a second operation a decade later. Adherence to the five Rs of secondary rhytidectomy will enable the plastic surgeon to safely restore youth and correct stigmata of primary face lift.

► Based on patient assessment and secondary procedures, the duration of a facelift may be between 7 and 10 years. It is expected that some patients will return for additional facial improvement. As the authors point out, the approach must address different components of rejuvenation in a secondary procedure. Attention needs to be paid to correcting improper skin or superficial musculo-aponeurotic system vectors from the primary procedure that contribute to the stigmata of a facelift. Volume restoration is more important, as these patients will be older and more likely to have facial volume loss because of skeletal changes and fat atrophy.

K. A. Gutowski, MD

Secondary Rhytidectomy: Comprehensive Review and Current Concepts

Rasko YM, Beale E, Rohrich RJ (Univ of Texas Southwestern Med Ctr, Dallas)
Plast Reconstr Surg 130:1370-1378, 2012

Background.—Secondary rhytidectomy procedures present an additional level of complexity in comparison with primary procedures. Patients may seek secondary rhytidectomy, in part, as a result of complications stemming from the initial procedure, because of the natural process of aging, or a combination of the two. The aim of this literature review was to examine the difference in patient characteristics, techniques, and challenges specific to secondary face lifts.

Methods.—A literature search was performed on secondary face-lift procedures using MEDLINE, PubMed, and Cochrane databases. Using the keywords "facelift," "face lift," "rhytidoplasty," and rhytidectomy combined with "secondary," "reoperation," "revision," and "multiple," an initial search was performed. Then, all abstracts were evaluated for relevance.

Results.—The search yielded 291 articles with these key terms. The articles were reviewed for relevance and, in total, 13 were identified specific to secondary rhytidectomy procedures. Six were retrospective studies and the rest were expert special topic articles.

Conclusions.—Although there are limited data specific to secondary rhytidectomy procedures, several important principles were evident from these retrospective reviews and editorial articles. It is important to assess whether the patient is exhibiting stigmata of the primary rhytidectomy procedure or natural signs of aging, such as volumetric deflation and recurring ptosis of previously lifted tissues. Accurate and systematic preoperative analysis is key for successful planning and execution of secondary rhytidectomy procedures.

▶ When evaluating a patient for a secondary rhytidectomy, issues to address include:

1. Prominent scars from the first procedure
   - In cases with wide scars, closure should be done with minimal tension.
   - When hypertrophic scars are present, early scar management should be started.
   - Inappropriately placed scars should be repositioned, if possible.
2. Hairline distortion
   - Pulling back the temporal hairline is a leading cause of "facelift stigmata"; therefore, anterior hairline incisions should be considered.
3. Ear deformities
   - If the tragus appears unnatural, a revision with skin defatting and minimal tension on the skin closure should be done.
   - Ear lobe distortion can be corrected by repositioning and a tension-free closure or by leaving the inferior portion of the ear lobe not attached to heal by secondary intention.
4. Cheek deformities
   - A lateral sweep can be corrected with flap repositioning.
   - Joker's lines can be improved with volume correction.
5. Neck deformities (sometimes not addressed at the first procedure)
   - An over- or undercorrected neck may require fat grafts or liposuction, respectively.
   - Platysmal bands should be corrected with a corset platysmaplasty (perhaps before the cheek superficial muscular aponeurotic system is manipulated to achieve a better reapproximation).
   - Partial caudal platysma transection can minimize recurrent bands.
6. Loss of facial volume
   - Volumetric correction with fat grafts should be used, as tissue repositioning and tightening alone will not improve cheek and perioral hollowing.

K. A. Gutowski, MD

Ultrasonically Assisted Face-Lift

de la Peña JA, Soto-Miranda MA, López-Salguero JF (Inst for Plastic Surgery, Huixquilucan, Mexico)

Aesthetic Plast Surg 36:780-787, 2012

Background.—The face-lift procedure is one of the most skillful interventions performed by plastic surgeons. Ultrasonic energy is used to elevate the facial skin flap, which allows for preservation of vascular, lymphatic, and nervous structures, thereby decreasing the morbidity associated with this procedure.

Methods.—A retrospective study to compare the outcomes of ultrasound and non-ultrasound-assisted face-lifts is reported. All the procedures were performed at the Institute for Plastic Surgery. Each group consisted of 104 patients. Statistical analysis was performed to determine differences between the groups.

Results.—The mean operating time was 4 h in the treatment group versus 4.2 h in the control group ($p > 0.05$). The incidence of hematoma formation was 0.96% in the treatment group versus 2.4% in the control group ($p < 0.05$). The incidence of flap necrosis was 0% in both groups. The duration of ecchymosis was 13 days in the experimental group versus 17.2 days in the control group ($p < 0.05$). The duration of postoperative swelling was 17.4 days in the treatment group versus 20.4 days in the control group ($p < 0.05$). As reported, 85% of patients in the treatment group were very satisfied, 14.42% were satisfied, 0% were mildly satisfied, and 0% were not satisfied. In the control group, 80.7% were very satisfied, 18.26% were satisfied, 0.96% were mildly satisfied, and 0% were not satisfied. According to Fisher's exact test, the p value for patient satisfaction exceeded 0.05%.

Conclusions.—The preservation of the blood and lymphatic vessels diminishes postoperative swelling and shortens the duration of ecchymosis considerably. The incidence of hematoma formation is lower than with a non-ultrasonic face-lift. This study failed to prove any statistically significant difference in operating time or patient satisfaction between the two groups.

▶ In this report, ultrasonic energy was safely used as a dissection tool to elevate the skin flaps while preserving vascularity. No claims were made about improved skin tightening compared with sharp skin flap elevation. Unfortunately, the details of the ultrasound energy level settings were not clearly explained.

K. A. Gutowski, MD

The eutrophic rhytidoplasty: Subdermal tunneling and minimal skin undermining

Daher M, Rodriguez Muñiz A (Interclinica-Centroplasticas, Rio de Janeiro, Brazil)

Eur J Plast Surg 36:87-94, 2013

Background.—Patients submitted to rhytidectomy usually relay their desire for briefer surgical procedures and a shorter post-operative period with faster recovery. In view of this, a technique in which the skin of the cervico-mandibular region is not undermined but only detached by blunt dissection was developed.

Methods.—A retrospective study of the senior author's experience in eutrophic rhytidoplasty (EUR), the technique proposed herein, for facial rejuvenation was conducted. Patients submitted to EUR over a 10-year period were included in this study. A total of 224 interventions were performed. The procedure consists of using subdermal tunneling, performed with a cannula along the neck region and the midface area (combined or not with liposuction in certain areas, as needed), thus preserving nervous and vascular connections. The conventional skin undermining is minimal, just 4 cm around the auricular pavilion. Data were collected from the patients' medical records at Interclínica—Centroplástica Clinic in Rio de Janeiro, Brazil.

Results.—Due to the skin eutrophic conditions, the operated patients, using the EUR technique, presented promising esthetical results. The mean rate of complications associated with the proposed technique was 1.7%. The author found that this technique offers very promising results, a fact evidenced by the lower rate of complications among patients submitted to it.

Conclusions.—The EUR is a reliable option for facial rejuvenation due to the fact that it is less invasive, with a low morbidity and rate of complications. Its surgical time is reduced by 50%, it has a shorter down-time, and yields natural results.

Level of Evidence.—Level IV, therapeutic study.

► This report describes a technique of subcutaneous facelift flap dissection with a 2-mm liposuction cannula (with or without suction as needed) beyond a conventional lateral skin flap elevation. It can be done using sedation and local anesthesia and includes standard superficial musculoaponeurotic system plication followed by skin redraping (which results in a decrease of fully undermined skin from 4 cm to 2 cm) and then closure. This is analogous to the lipoabdominoplasty concept of tunnel undermining with a liposuction cannula to minimize damage to abdominal flap neurovascular bundles. In the face, it may be useful in cases in which poor cutaneous blood perfusion may be present, such as in heavy smokers. Unfortunately, the authors did not present enough before and after pictures to truly judge the effectiveness of this method.

K. A. Gutowski, MD

Thirteen Years of Experience With the Endoscopic Midface Lift

Saltz R, Ohana B (Private Practice in Salt Lake City, UT; Private Practice in Rio de Janeiro, Brazil)

Aesthet Surg J 32:927-936, 2012

Background.—Numerous techniques have been used to rejuvenate the aging midface. The Endotine midface technique involves an endoscopic temporal approach, including midface dissection and malar suspension with fixation. The Endotine device (Microaire, Charlottesville, Virginia) eliminates the intraoral incision and use of sutures, enabling multipoint fixation and fast, simple adjustability for optimal control of midface elevation and volume.

Objectives.—The authors describe their preferred technique for the endoscopic midface lift and summarize their 13 years of experience.

Methods.—A retrospective chart review was conducted of 183 patients who underwent endoscopic midface surgery. Patients treated from 1998 to 2003 received direct needle fixation (n = 95). Those treated later underwent fixation with the Endotine device (n = 88).

Results.—Most (90%) of the patient population was female, and the average age at the time of surgery was 46 years (range, 39-54 years). Needle fixation was used in 95 patients and Endotine fixation in 88. The average follow-up period was 7 years. The authors have observed many improvements in outcomes since the introduction of the Endotine device into their practice. These include reduced swelling and bruising, more symmetric elevation of the malar fat pad, mild improvement of tear trough deformity, softening of the nasolabial folds, and, in some cases, decreased "jowling." The asymmetry often associated with direct needle fixation has decreased, and no skin dimpling has occurred. Through their experience, the authors' preferred technique has become the temporal-only approach with Endotine fixation.

Conclusions.—The Endotine midface suspension device enhances soft-tissue fixation, provides simple adjustability for optimal elevation and projection, and maintains mechanical fixation until biologic fixation becomes adequate. The 5 tines provide multiple points of contact for secure soft-tissue fixation. Elevation forces are evenly distributed over a wide area, which eliminates skin irregularities. Insertion and deployment are accomplished easily through temporal incision.

▶ Midface lifts can result in improved facial rejuvenation that cannot always be achieved with a lateral cheek facelift alone. However, the evolution of facial volume replacement with fillers and fat may have resulted in less surgical corrections of the midface. The endoscopic approach to the midface avoids potential complications involving the lower eyelid but does require a more complex dissection, which puts the temporal branch of the facial nerve at risk (in this series, about half of the patients had a temporary nerve weakness). Another criticism of the endoscopic approach is that it does not always achieve predictable results. Based on long-term follow-up, it now seems that the use of a bioabsorbable fixation system (Endotine) can make the procedure easier with a lower revision rate. Proper patient selection for an isolated midface lift should exclude older patients with facial skin excess who would be better served with a full facelift, and those with significant facial volume loss.

K. A. Gutowski, MD

Complications of Browlift Techniques: A Systematic Review

Byun S, Mukovozov I, Farrokhyar F, et al (McMaster Univ, Hamilton, Ontario, Canada; Univ of Toronto, Ontario, Canada)

Aesthet Surg J 33:189-200, 2013

Background.—There is ongoing debate over which surgical technique is the safest for brow elevation.

Objectives.—The authors outline complication rates for a variety of open and endoscopic browlift techniques based on the results of a literature review.

Methods.—The following databases were searched to capture relevant studies: MEDLINE, EMBASE, CINAHL, LILACS, Web of Science, Cochrane Libraries, controlled-trials.com, and clinicaltrials.gov. Eighty-two studies met the inclusion criteria. Assuming between-study heterogeneity due to the limitations and biases inherent to case series, a random-effects model was used to calculate weighted proportions. Pooled weighted proportions with 95% confidence intervals were determined.

Results.—All open and endoscopic procedures are associated with a variety of complications. Unacceptable scarring and paresthesia are the most common complications among all surgical browlifts. For anterior hairline incision with subcutaneous dissection, alopecia occurred in 8.5% of patients, paresthesia in 5.4%, unacceptable scarring in 2.1%, and skin necrosis in 1.8%. For coronal incision with subgaleal dissection, unacceptable scarring occurred in 3.6% of patients, hematoma in 0.5%, and infection in 0.2%. Endoscopic techniques with subperiosteal dissection had the highest complication rates: 6.2% for paresthesia, 3.6% for asymmetry, 3.0% for alopecia, and 2.7% for lagophthalmos.

Conclusions.—Although complication rates vary with respect to incision site and plane of dissection, endoscopic techniques are associated with a larger variety of complications than open approaches. The findings should be interpreted with caution due to the limitations inherent to a case series. A well-designed comparative study is needed to evaluate the "true" rate of complications among the various browlift techniques.

► Although all browlifts (open and endoscopic) have risks of complications, this review shows that more seem to occur with endoscopic techniques. However, other factors in the clinical decision-making process of choosing the technique were not addressed. These results need to be incorporated into the full risk-to-benefit profile (which includes brow position, longevity of outcomes, costs, recovery time, and standardized quality-of-life and patient-reported outcomes measurements). Perhaps a well-designed comparative study will give a better understanding of the complications of browlifting procedures.

K. A. Gutowski, MD

Endoscopic forehead lift in patients with male pattern baldness

Shipchandler TZ, Sultan B, Byrne PJ (Indiana Univ School of Medicine, Indianapolis; Johns Hopkins Univ School of Medicine, Baltimore, MD)
Am J Otolaryngol 33:519-522, 2012

Purpose.—The presence of male pattern baldness poses a significant challenge when attempting to optimize treatment of the upper third of the face. The purpose of this study is to demonstrate and discuss results of the endoscopic forehead lift in patients with male pattern baldness.

Materials and Methods.—This was a retrospective case series done in an academic medical center. Eleven patients with male pattern baldness (Norwood class IV–VII) underwent endoscopic forehead lift for forehead creases and brow ptosis.

Results.—All patients achieved smoothing of the forehead and elevation of the brow with no scalp anesthesia at 1 month postoperatively. All patients were pleased with the healing of their incisions in midline, paramedian, and temporal regions. Alloplastic fixation devices used were visible postoperatively in 2 patients initially.

Conclusions.—The endoscopic forehead lift is a suitable approach for treating the upper third of the face in the presence of male pattern baldness. The use of alloplastic fixation devices may be used in this patient population, but other fixation methods should be considered.

▶ Many options exist for male forehead and brow lifts, each with its own advantages and disadvantages. The endoscopic approach, with proper incision orientation in the paramedian and temporal areas (the midline incision described in this series is not needed), will generally yield minimal scars even in areas of hair loss. Even with use of the Endotine absorbable fixation device, the incisions are small enough to not be noticeable. However, as men tend to have heavier brows and stronger brow depressor muscle forces, endoscopic techniques don't always provide lasting results; therefore, proper patient education and expectations need to be considered.

K. A. Gutowski, MD

Eyelid

Augmentation Blepharoplasty: A Review of 500 Consecutive Patients

Tonnard PL, Verpaele AM, Zeltzer AA (Gent Univ Hosp, Belgium; Brussels Univ Hosp, Belgium)
Aesthet Surg J 33:341-352, 2013

Background.—Volume loss in the upper and lower eyelids and in the malar area is now considered a major component of periorbital aging. As classical resection blepharoplasty does not address this loss, filling procedures are becoming increasingly common.

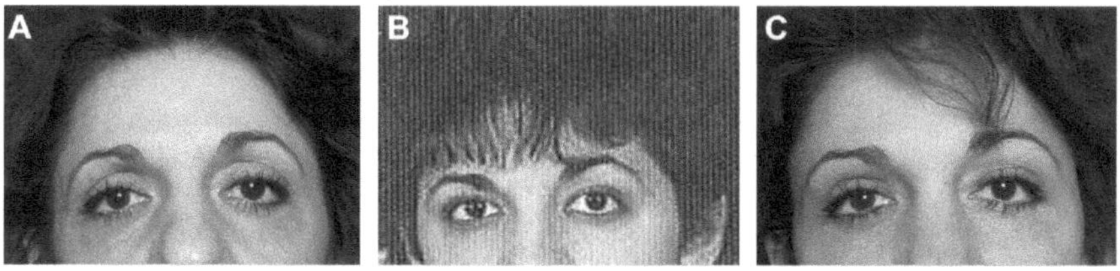

FIGURE 5.—(A) This 46-year-old woman presented for total facial rejuvenation. Her periorbital area shows hollowing of the medial part of the upper eyelid and a slight descent in the tail of the eyebrow. The lower eyelid shows demarcation of the eyelid-cheek junction and atrophy of the malar region, especially in the anterior part. (B) A picture of the same patient taken at age 25 years shows full and crisp upper eyelids and full malar regions without eyelid-cheek demarcation. (C) Two years after extended minimal-access cranial suspension lift, temporal lift, rhinoplasty, fat grafting of the nasolabial folds (3 mL per side) and marionette grooves (2.5 mL on the right side; 3 mL on the left), and augmentation blepharoplasty. In the upper eyelid, 2.5 mL of fat was grafted on each side and no skin was resected. In the lower eyelid area, 10 mL of fat was grafted in the orbitomalar area with additional pinch skin blepharoplasty. (Reprinted from Tonnard PL, Verpaele AM, Zeltzer AA. Augmentation blepharoplasty: a review of 500 consecutive patients. *Aesthet Surg J*. 2013;33:341-352, © 2013, Aesthetic Surgery Journal.)

Objectives.—The authors present their experience with periorbital fat grafting in conjunction with routine blepharoplasty to address periorbital aging.

Methods.—Outcomes were retrospectively reviewed for 500 consecutive patients who underwent blepharoplasty in conjunction with the authors' periorbital augmentation technique from January 2008 to September 2011. The augmentation technique was a fine particle fat (microfat) grafting procedure that involved the use of small-diameter cannulae for transfer of autologous fat to the medial part of the upper eyelid, the orbitomalar groove, and the malar area.

Results.—Clinical evaluation and review of patient photographs revealed favorable, natural-looking, and long-lasting improvement of the treated areas. Shortcomings of classical resection blepharoplasty, such as hollowing of the upper eyelids, incomplete blending of the eyelid-cheek junction, and persistent deflation of the midface, were avoided; the full and crisp aspect of the upper and lower eyelids seen at a younger age was regained; and the technique was not associated with the complications seen in an earlier patient series. No major complications occurred. Minor complications included bruising and swelling.

Conclusions.—Augmentation of the upper and lower eyelids through microfat grafting can be a useful alternative to existing blepharoplasty techniques. This study documents very natural and pleasing results that avoid the shortcomings of classical resection. Microfat grafting appears to be a valuable and safe alternative to complicated, difficult, and potentially dangerous eyelid and midface rejuvenation techniques (Fig 5).

▶ This is an interesting, albeit noncontrolled, retrospective clinical study based on the evolving experiences of 3 Belgian plastic surgeons. By and large the photos presented tend to document the authors' technique. I was intrigued, in one case, by the inclusion of a photograph of a patient at a much younger age

(Fig 5) and the suggestion by the authors that all patients bring such photographs with them to allow the surgeon to plan appropriate periorbital rejuvenation. The most obvious benefits seem to be in the medial region of the upper eyelid and the malar–orbital junction. However, it is somewhat difficult to separate the results in the periorbital regions from that presented from the effects of more global facial surgery in the photos presented. Finally, as in most current thoughts about aesthetic surgery, less is better than more, and correction of aging and cosmetic deformity requires a judicious blend of excision and addition of appropriate tissue.

S. H. Miller, MD

Evaluation of Orbicularis Oculi Muscle Stripping on the Cosmetic Outcome of Upper Lid Blepharoplasty: A Randomized, Controlled Study

Lopiccolo MC, Mahmoud BH, Liu A, et al (Henry Ford Hosp, Detroit, MI; et al)
Dermatol Surg 39:739-743, 2013

Background.—Many variations in the surgical treatment of upper eyelid blepharoplasty have been described, including orbicularis oculi muscle stripping. There is no evidence in the literature to support the efficacy of this technique in improving the aesthetic results of the procedure.

Objectives.—To conduct a single-blind, randomized, controlled, split-face pilot study to evaluate the effects of orbicularis oculi muscle stripping on upper lid blepharoplasty.

Methods.—Ten subjects were randomized to receive upper lid blepharoplasty with orbicularis oculi muscle stripping on one side and skin-only blepharoplasty on the other. Patients and two blinded physicians evaluated the aesthetics of the eyelids at 1-, 3-, and 17-month follow-up visits.

Results.—Blinded physician evaluation failed to show a difference in the overall cosmetic appearance of the eyelids between the control and treatment sides at any time point. Analysis of the composite of all patient scores showed a trend favoring the control side at 3 months ($p = .28$) and the treatment side at 17 months ($p = .50$), but neither difference was significant.

Conclusion.—Based on the data from this pilot study, orbicularis oculi muscle stripping appears to have no affect on the aesthetic outcome of upper lid blepharoplasty.

▶ Although this study failed to find an advantage with orbicularis oculi resection compared with no resection, only a 2- to 4-mm-wide strip of muscle was removed. Also, fat resection was not done in any of the cases. Perhaps a better-designed study would be more useful to answer the question of muscle resection in upper lid blepharoplasty.

K. A. Gutowski, MD

A New Approach: Resection and Suture of Orbicularis Oculi Muscle to Define the Upper Eyelid Fold and Correct Asymmetries

Bas CT, Pérez-Guisado J (Sara Moncada Clinic, Providencia, Chile; Reina Sofía Univ Hosp, Córdoba, Spain)
Aesthetic Plast Surg 37:46-50, 2013

Upper-eyelid blepharoplasty is a very common procedure in aesthetic plastic surgery. Among all the literature in favor of orbicularis muscle resection, there are no commentaries associated with orbicularis muscle suture and its convenience. This article discusses a new approach: independent resection of the orbicularis oculi muscle similar in size to the resected skin and the subsequent suture of the orbicularis muscle after its resection. This results in a fine reconstruction of the upper-eyelid crease, achieves a good definition of this anatomical structure, and allows correction of asymmetries with the contralateral upper eyelid. The results obtained (98% of patients satisfied) and no complications with this procedure make it a safe alternative for upper blepharoplasty.

Level of Evidence IV.—This journal requires that authors assign a level of evidence to each article. For a full description of these Evidence-Based Medicine ratings, please refer to the Table of Contents or the online Instructions to Authors www.springer.com/00266.

▶ Most surgeons use a single layer closure of the skin (which may include the underlying orbicularis oculi muscle) in upper blepharoplasties. This technique uses a separate suture for muscle reapproximation in an attempt to provide better eyelid fold definition. Although the results are good, they do not seem any better than those of single layer skin closure.

K. A. Gutowski, MD

A New Approach: Resection and Suture of Orbicularis Oculi Muscle to Define the Upper Eyelid Fold and Correct Asymmetries

Bas CT, Pérez-Guisado J (Sara Moncada Clinic, Providencia, Santiago de Chile; Reina Sofía Univ Hosp, Córdoba, Spain)
Aesthetic Plast Surg 37:46-50, 2013

Upper-eyelid blepharoplasty is a very common procedure in aesthetic plastic surgery. Among all the literature in favor of orbicularis muscle resection, there are no commentaries associated with orbicularis muscle suture and its convenience. This article discusses a new approach: independent resection of the orbicularis oculi muscle similar in size to the resected skin and the subsequent suture of the orbicularis muscle after its resection. This results in a fine reconstruction of the upper-eyelid crease, achieves a good definition of this anatomical structure, and allows correction of asymmetries with the contralateral upper eyelid. The results obtained (98% of patients satisfied) and no complications with this procedure make it a safe alternative for upper blepharoplasty.

Level of Evidence IV.—This journal requires that authors assign a level of evidence to each article. For a full description of these Evidence-Based Medicine ratings, please refer to the Table of Contents or the online Instructions to Authors www.springer.com/00266.

▶ To resect or not to resect? To suture or not to suture? It is very difficult to know whether the authors' technique is superior to that described by those who believe that no resection is necessary or whether resection of the amount of muscle should be equal or different from the amount of skin resected. Is it necessary to suture the orbicularis oculi or should we allow it to heal naturally after the skin edges are coapted? Unfortunately, this article does little to answer the questions, other than to promote the authors' procedure. The one report that attempted to study whether resection of the muscle mattered in the end showed an initial difference, but in the long term whether the muscle was resected or not did not seem to matter.[1] Is it possible that whether or not one sutures the muscle will make little or no difference in the long-term end result?

S. H. Miller, MD

Reference

1. Damasceno RW, Cariello NJ, Cardoso EB, Viana GA, Osaki MH. Upper blepharoplasty with or without resection of the orbicularis oculi muscle: a randomized double-blind left-right study. *Ophthal Plast Reconstr Surg*. 2011;27:195-197.

Nose

What Motivates Secondary Rhinoplasty? A Study of 150 Consecutive Patients

Constantian MB (Univ of Wisconsin; Nashua, NH)
Plast Reconstr Surg 130:667-678, 2012

Background.—There is little evidence-based information on secondary rhinoplasty patient motivations for surgery, satisfaction, or revision rates.

Methods.—The charts of 150 consecutive patients (121 women and 29 men) who underwent secondary rhinoplasty between July of 2007 and October of 2008 were reviewed; preoperative deformity severity was graded from 1 to 5. The patients' primary reasons for surgery, patient and surgeon satisfaction, and postoperative depression or body dysmorphic disorder were tallied.

Results.—The average number of prior operations was 3.6. The most commonly expressed reason (41 percent) for undergoing revision was the development of a new deformity after the primary rhinoplasty. Those patients also had the most severe preoperative deformities ($p < 0.02$). Other motivations were failure to correct the original deformity (33 percent), an intolerable perceived loss of personal, familial, or ethnic characteristics (15 percent), the desire for further improvement in an already

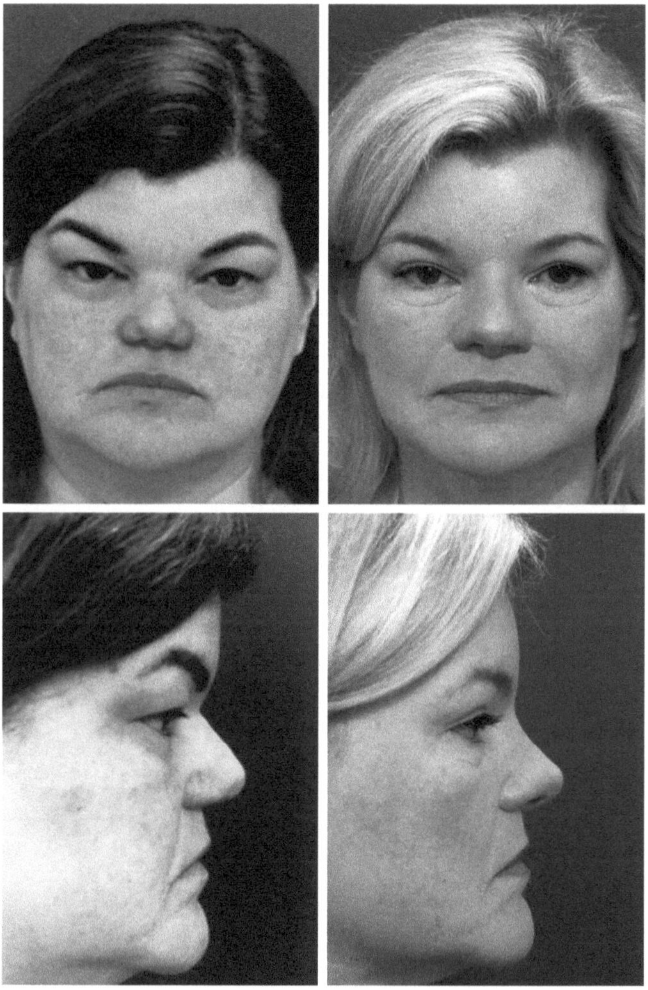

FIGURE 1.—Case 1. A 42-year-old secondary patient presented with a new postoperative deformity. She had undergone placement of a silicone implant that failed to correct her airway or contour. Reconstruction involved rib cartilage dorsal, alar wall, columellar, and tip grafts; alar rim excisions; and a coronal brow lift. (*Above, left*) Preoperative frontal view. (*Above, right*) Postoperative frontal view at 4 years. (*Below, left*) Preoperative lateral view. (*Below, right*) Postoperative lateral view at 4 years. (Reprinted from Constantian MB. What motivates secondary rhinoplasty? A study of 150 consecutive patients. *Plast Reconstr Surg*. 2012;130:667-678, the American Society of Plastic Surgeons.)

acceptable result (10 percent), and a new or unrelieved airway obstruction (1 percent). Ninety-seven percent of patients were happy with their outcomes. Forty patients (27 percent) were depressed before surgery and three (2 percent) displayed evidence of body dysmorphic disorder postoperatively. The depressed and dysmorphic patients did not have worse deformities than those who were not depressed postoperatively ($p < 0.8695$).

Conclusions.—Most secondary rhinoplasty patients have motivations similar to those of our other reconstructive patients and will be pleased with their surgical outcomes. The most severe preoperative deformities were iatrogenic. The unhappy postoperative patients, including those with body dysmorphic disorder, did not have more severe preoperative deformities than the others (i.e., their deformities alone did not justify their unhappiness) (Fig 1).

▶ This is an interesting self-directed analysis of the results the author achieved following secondary rhinoplasty. He is generally recognized as a master rhinoplastic surgeon, and his self-improvement efforts are worthy of emulation by all surgeons involved in clinical practice. I am happy to see that he reported on a series of consecutive patients and that he achieved such a high level of satisfaction after secondary surgery. It is of interest that almost 70% of the patients operated on were the patients of other surgeons as opposed to the other 30%, who were secondary (tertiary) revisions on his own patients. I am concerned about the average number of revisions per patient being 3.6 (range 1–8) and not knowing whether the outcomes varied with the number of revisions. I also find myself concerned with the high number of demanding and depressed patients and wonder if he sought preoperative assistance from a mental health worker in some or any of these patients. Is the patient in Fig 1 really a new deformity or an inappropriately executed procedure in the first place? Finally, lest we forget, the large volume of rhinoplasty cases performed by this surgeon very likely is a major factor in his good results and may not be generalizable to all plastic surgeons.

S. H. Miller, MD

The Use of Short Spreader Grafts in Rhinoplasty for Patients with Thick Nasal Skin

Grigoryants V, Baroni A (Plastic and Reconstructive Surgery, Glendale, CA)
Aesthetic Plast Surg 37:516-520, 2013

Background.—Thick nasal skin presents a challenge in rhinoplasty. Conventional spreader grafts in patients with thick nasal skin may result in an undesirable widening of the lower half of the nose where the nasal skin is thick. The use of short spreader grafts was evaluated in patients with thick nasal skin.

Methods.—For this study, 32 patients underwent closed rhinoplasty in which short spreader grafts were used. The spreader graft was 1 to 2 cm long and extended only to the transition of thin and thick nasal skin. The patients were followed for more than 1 year postoperatively.

Results.—Aesthetic improvement was observed in all the patients. Nasal airway patency was improved or maintained in 94% of the patients.

Conclusions.—Short spreader grafts effectively restore or maintain the internal nasal valve area after dorsal hump reduction while allowing for more aggressive narrowing of the lower part of the nose where nasal skin is thick.

Level of Evidence.—IV This journal requires that authors assign a level of evidence to each article. For a full description of these Evidence-Based Medicine ratings, please refer to the Table of Contents or the online Instructions to Authors www.springer.com/00266.

▶ Spreader grafts traditionally have been described as 30 to 35 mm long and as useful in improving internal valve function, correcting dorsal irregularities, and preventing deformity after dorsal hump reduction. However, in patients with thick nasal skin, conventional spreader grafts that extend to the caudal end of the septum may cause undesirable lower nasal widening or limit the surgeon's ability to narrow a wide tip. In this patient series, the spreader grafts did not extend to the area of thick nasal skin but were designed shorter, yet wide enough to lateralize the upper lateral cartilages adequately and support the mid-nasal vault. Although most patients had an improved nasal airway after surgery, care must be taken when drawing conclusions about the role of the short spreader grafts alone in the functional outcome, because septoplasty was performed in most of the patients and turbinate reduction was done in all the patients (which could account for the improved results).

K. A. Gutowski, MD

Liposuction, Fat Transfer, and Tissue Fillers

Autologous Fat Transfer for Face Rejuvenation with Tumescent Technique Fat Harvesting and Saline Washing: A Report of 215 Cases

Rusciani Scorza A, Rusciani Scorza L, Troccola A, et al (Univ of Rome 'La Sapienza', Italy; et al)

Dermatology 224:244-250, 2012

Various materials have been used for tissue augmentation and for the treatment of rhytids. Autologous fat transfer (AFT) is considered ideal regarding biocompatibility and patient concerns. This study was performed on a series of 215 female patients for face rejuvenation with tumescent technique fat harvesting and saline washing. The study was based on two AFT procedures for each patient. Second treatment was performed at least 1 month after the first operation. Their mean age was 55.5 ± 2.1 years. High-definition photographs in five standard views, front (n = 1), side (n = 2) and oblique of 3/4 (n = 2), were taken for the preoperative morphological study. Aesthetic outcomes were evaluated by the operating surgeon, the patient and an independent dermatologist. Outcomes were evaluated by comparing the preoperative photographs with those taken 1 month after the first procedure and at the end of the 1-year follow-up period. At 12 months all the patients except one noted an improvement. Of these 85.6% (184 patients) were satisfied with the treatment. The operating surgeon and the independent observer noted respectively a sufficient correction in 88.8 and 95.3%. AFT was considered painless by 94.9% and slightly painful by 5.1% of subjects. Fat tissue harvesting by tumescent anesthesia and purification with saline washing enable adipocyte viability to be preserved throughout the procedure and to perform the treatment under local anesthesia.

▶ This large series of facial fat-graft patients suggests that centrifugation and more complex fat preparation techniques may not be needed to assure good clinical results. Simple saline washes of the aspirated fat may be adequate. Unfortunately, the authors were not very detailed in their technique description, stating only: "The adipose tissue is washed with saline to remove all blood and cell elements, and left to stand; 10–12 washes yield a layer of saline and a supernatant predominantly comprised of bright yellow adipocytes and growth factors. This procedure is done in the same 10 ml Luer lock syringe used during fat harvesting. The piston is never removed from the harvesting syringe during washing to avoid tissue exposure to air." We are left unsure as to how much volume to use for the washes and how long to let the fat stand and separate. The authors also did not describe if they fill the facial soft tissue to the desired amount of volume or if they "overfill" by some amount to account for fat graft loss. It seems that some of these details may need to be worked out by each surgeon.

K. A. Gutowski, MD

Supplementing Fat Grafts with Adipose Stromal Cells for Cosmetic Facial Contouring

Li J, Gao J, Cha P, et al (Southern Med Univ, Guangzhou, China)

Dermatol Surg 39:449-456, 2013

Background.—Numerous methods have been proposed to enhance the survival of fat grafts, but no definitive treatment is available. Stromal vascular fraction (SVF)-assisted cell therapy offers new perspectives for improving fat graft survival.

Objectives.—To determine whether SVF supplementation could improve graft retention in patients undergoing autologous fat grafting for cosmetic improvement of facial contour.

Methods.—We retrospectively analyzed data from 38 women who underwent fat transplantation with SVF ($n = 26$) or fat grafting alone ($n = 12$) between October 2010 and January 2012. Each patient underwent computed tomography, and photographs were taken before and 6 months after surgery. The Philips Extended Brilliance Workspace was used for analysis of volume augmentation.

Results.—All patients showed cosmetic improvements, but the degree varied. No complications were evidenced during follow-up. Fat survival was higher with SVF (64.8 ± 10.2%) than fat grafting alone (46.4 ± 9.3%) ($p < .01$). SVF supplementation resulted in better clinical improvement than fat grafting alone.

Conclusion.—Supplementing fat grafts with SVF for cosmetic facial contouring can improve the survival of fat grafts over fat grafting alone and provides satisfactory outcomes without major complications. Autologous fat grafting has been used for various cosmetic treatments and difficult reconstructive indications such as temporal depression, wrinkles of nasolabial folds, and hemifacial atrophy, with no incisional scar or complications associated with foreign materials, although problems such as a low rate of graft survival because of early resorption remain. (Aesthet Plast Surg, 14, 1990 and 127) Despite many innovations to overcome these problems, (Dermatol Surg, 26, 2000 and 1159); (Ann Plast Surg, 60, 2008 and 594); (Dermatol Surg, 27, 2001 and 819); (Dermatol Surg, 28, 2002 and 987) we lack a definitive method of fat processing that ensures maximal graft take and viability. (Plast Reconstr Surg, 115, 2005 and 197); (Dermatol Surg, 37, 2011 and 619).

▶ Stromal vascular fraction (SVF) contains cells consisting of adipose tissue–derived stem cells, endothelial progenitor cells, hematopoietic progenitors, T cells, and anti-inflammatory cells. SVF acts as the main player in adipogenesis and angiogenesis in the adipose repair process by not only differentiating into adipocytes or vascular endothelial cells, but also releasing angiogenic growth factors. In this study, the SVF processing took about 60 minutes and required a multistep process of filtration, resuspension, incubation, and cell washing (a process that would require proper regulatory approval under current US Food and Drug Administration guidelines). The results of this well-designed study suggest that there may be a role for SVF supplementation of fat grafts in the near future. For clinical applications to be widespread, the cell processing will need to be simplified and regulatory issues addressed.

K. A. Gutowski, MD

Hyaluronic Acid Filler Injections for Tear-Trough Deformity: Injection Technique and High-Frequency Ultrasound Follow-up Evaluation

De Pasquale A, Russa G, Pulvirenti M, et al ("San Vincenzo" Hosp, Taormina, Sicily, Italy; "Civico- G.DI Cristina-Benfratelli" Hosp, Palermo, Sicily, Italy; Private Practice, Palermo, Sicily, Italy; et al)
Aesthetic Plast Surg 37:587-591, 2013

This study aimed to describe the technique used by the authors in treating tear-trough deformity and to illustrate the effectiveness of high-frequency diagnostic ultrasound in the assessment of dermal filler longevity. In this consecutive interventional nonrandomized case series, 22 patients (18 women and 4 men) were evaluated. They ranged in age from 29 to 65 years (mean, 46.59 years ± 10.0 years). The patients were given multiple hyaluronic acid injections in the tear-trough area between 2009 and 2011. The injected areas then were evaluated with sonographic scans during the follow-up period. All the patients were examined preoperatively,

7 days after injection, then after 1, 6, and 12 months, and finally once a year. Pre- and postoperative photographs using standard positioning and lighting were taken as well as high-frequency ultrasound scans using a 15-MHz scanner with an axial resolution of 15 mm. The injection technique consisted of three to five injections perpendicular to the skin. These were administered just under the orbital rim, creating three column-shaped hyaluronic acid deposits deep in the orbicularis oculi muscle, from 0.2 mm to 0.5 mm below the orbital rim. Approximately 0.1 ml—0.3 ml was injected at a time. This technique creates a deep scaffolding that can fill the orbital hollow. The amount of filler used in each area ranged from 0.1 ml to 0.3 ml (mean, 0.267 ml ± 0.128 ml), whereas the mean filler quantity in each eyelid was 0.45 ml ± 0.14 ml. During the follow-up visit 1 week after the treatment, 21 patients (90%) required a second series of injections either in the exact same areas or right next to the injected area to obtain a smoother appearance of the skin surface. During the sonographer examination, it was always possible to identify and measure the filler at the site of the injection.

Level of Evidence IV.—This journal requires that authors assign a level of evidence to each article. For a full description of these Evidence-Based Medicine ratings, please refer to the Table of Contents or the online Instructions to Authors www.springer.com/00266.

▶ Periorbital soft tissue filler injections around the orbit require a higher level of skill than most other facial areas. The thin skin and thin layer of subcutaneous tissue make this region less forgiving with visible product irregularities and prolonged edema as a consequence. Hyaluronic acids (HA) seem to be the best choice of filler in this area, as they are somewhat moldable and soft and can be reversed with hyaluronidase. Using ultrasound imaging, the authors demonstrated that their technique— 3 to 5 injection points per tear trough, injection perpendicular to the skin, HA placement just below the orbital rim, 0.1 to 0.3 mL per an injection point, placing a column of HA from the periosteum to orbicularis muscle, gentle massage for smoothing of the HA, and follow-up injection at 1 week if needed—gives lasting results with good aesthetic outcomes.

K. A. Gutowski, MD

A Decade of Experience with Injectable Poly-L-Lactic Acid: A Focus on Safety

Bartus C, William Hanke C, Daro-Kaftan E (Advanced Dermatology Associates, Allentown, PA; Laser and Skin Surgery Ctr of Indiana, Carmel; Peloton Advantage, Parsippany, NJ)

Dermatol Surg 39:698-705, 2013

Background.—Injectable poly-L-lactic acid (PLLA) is a biodegradable synthetic polymer device that stimulates collagen production, leading to gradual volume restoration. It has been used worldwide for more than a decade to treat the lines and wrinkles of the aging face and in individuals with the human immunodeficiency virus for treatment of facial lipoatrophy.

Objective.—To provide an overview of the experience with injectable PLLA in Europe and the United States and the practices that have improved product use.

Materials and Methods.—A review of the literature was conducted, and the authors' clinical experience was included detailing the evolution of the use of injectable PLLA for facial restoration.

Results.—Although relatively high rates of nodule and papule formation were reported during early use of injectable PLLA, updated methods have led to better safety and efficacy, including patient selection, preparation, and instruction; product preparation; timing of injections and avoidance of overcorrection; an updated understanding of the anatomy of the aging face; and site-specific injection techniques.

Conclusion.—Important lessons have been learned that have enhanced the safety and efficacy of injectable PLLA and have made it a desirable product for restoring facial volume.

▶ After a better understanding of the use of poly-L-lactic acid (Sculptra), there seem to be fewer adverse events and better patient outcomes. The ability of this product to allow for diffuse facial injections makes it a good choice for correction of global facial volume loss seen in aging. This article is worth reviewing to understand the specific injection techniques for different facial zones.

K. A. Gutowski, MD

Techniques for the Optimization of Facial and Nonfacial Volumization with Injectable Poly-L-lactic Acid

Paul Lorenc Z (Lorenc Aesthetic Plastic Surgery Ctr, NY)

Aesthetic Plast Surg 36:1222-1229, 2012

With the recognition of the key role of volume loss in the facial aging process, injectable dermal fillers and volumizers have become increasingly important treatment options for recontouring and rejuvenating the aging face. While replacement fillers effectively correct individual lines and wrinkles, volumizing agents that replace collagen provide a longer-lasting, volume-based alternative. Poly-L-lactic acid (PLLA) has been shown to increase dermal thickness and volume for up to 2 years and beyond. Although early clinical use of this agent in patients with HIV-associated facial lipoatrophy was associated with a significant rate of nodule or papule formation, subsequent experience has helped define the proper reconstitution volumes and injection techniques for optimizing results and minimizing nodule/papule formation. While injectable PLLA has been used successfully for rejuvenation of most facial areas, increasing experience suggests that it is a versatile agent capable of providing aesthetic enhancement in multiple areas of the body, including the dorsum of the hands, the décolleté, the neck, the buttocks, the medial ankles, and acne scars. Although the current published experience in these areas is limited, further studies and clinical use of injectable PLLA will clarify the potential of this agent as a minimally invasive alternative and/or adjunct to surgery for restoring volume loss in multiple anatomic areas.

Level of Evidence V.—This journal requires that authors assign a level of evidence to each article. For a full description of these Evidence-Based Medicine ratings, please refer to the Table of Contents or the online Instructions to Authors www.springer.com/00266.

▶ The initially approved indication for poly-L-lactic acid (PLLA, Sculptra) was treatment of human immunodeficiency virus—associated lipoatrophy. It is now used for aesthetic indications, including improvement of volume deficits in the nasolabial and malar regions, temples, cheeks, preauricular regions, perioral commissures, and jawline. It is also used off label to treat a variety of nonfacial areas, including the dorsum of the hands, décolleté, neck, postsurgical irregularities, and acne scars. The authors' recommendations on dilution methods and injection techniques should be considered by all who use PLLA in their practice. Briefly, the PLLA should be reconstituted to at least a total of 9 mL (5 mL sterile water for injection + 4 mL lidocaine 1% or lidocaine 1% and epinephrine 1:100 000) at least 24 hours before use (but 2–3 days may be better). The injection plane should be supraperiosteal for malar, temporal, pyriform, and mandibular areas and subcutaneous for the lower midface. Treatment of the periorbital area is not currently recommended because of an increased risk of papules and nodules in this area.

K. A. Gutowski, MD

Trunk, Genitalia, and Extremities

A Multivariate Regression Analysis of Panniculectomy Outcomes: Does Plastic Surgery Training Matter?

Mioton LM, Buck DW II, Gart MS, et al (Northwestern Univ, Chicago, IL)
Plast Reconstr Surg 131:604e-612e, 2013

Background.—Panniculectomy can improve quality of life in morbidly obese patients, but its functional benefits are counterbalanced by relatively high complication rates. The authors endeavored to determine the impact of plastic surgery training on panniculectomy outcomes.

Methods.—A retrospective review was performed of the prospectively maintained American College of Surgeons National Surgical Quality Improvement Program database for all patients undergoing panniculectomy from 2006 to 2010. Patient demographic details, surgeon specialty training, and 30-day outcomes were assessed.

Results.—A total of 954 panniculectomies meeting inclusion criteria were identified. Plastic surgeons performed 694 (72.7 percent) of the procedures, and 260 (27.3 percent) were performed by nonplastic surgeons. Nonplastic surgeons had significantly higher rates of overall complications (23.08 percent versus 8.65 percent; $p < 0.001$) and wound infections (12.69 percent versus 5.33 percent; $p < 0.001$) than plastic surgeons. Average operative time for plastic surgeons was significantly longer than that for nonplastic surgeons (3.00 ± 1.48 hours versus 1.88 ± 0.93 hours; $p < 0.001$). Risk-adjusted multivariate regression showed that undergoing a panniculectomy by a nonplastic surgeon was a significant predictor of overall postoperative complications (odds ratio, 2.09; 95 percent CI, 1.35 to 3.23) and wound infection (odds ratio, 1.73; 95 percent CI, 1.004 to 2.98). Subgroup analysis of propensity-matched samples supported this finding.

Conclusion.—Multivariate regression analysis of National Surgical Quality Improvement Program data showed that panniculectomy performed by plastic surgeons results in lower rates of overall postoperative complications compared with that performed by nonplastic surgeons.

▶ It may not be surprising that panniculectomy outcomes are better when the procedure is done by plastic surgeons. These findings should be disseminated to other surgeons to ensure that patients have access to the proper surgical specialist when a panniculectomy is planned.

K. A. Gutowski, MD

Evaluation of the Weight Loss Patient Presenting for Plastic Surgery Consultation

Bossert RP, Peter Rubin J (Univ of Pittsburgh School of Medicine, PA)
Plast Reconstr Surg 130:1361-1369, 2012

Patients presenting for plastic surgery consultation after massive weight loss require a thorough preoperative evaluation that takes into account the complex medical and psychosocial issues associated with obesity. A number of factors must be considered, including type of weight loss procedure, nutritional deficiencies, body mass index at the time of consultation, and unresolved cardiovascular and pulmonary problems. This assessment will help identify issues requiring more detailed evaluation, provide an accurate risk profile, allow for optimization of active disease states before surgery, and increase patient safety.

▶ Patients with massive weight loss, particularly those presenting after bariatric surgery, have unique issues that should be addressed before considering surgical body contouring. The recommendations described are particularly useful for plastic surgeons whose patients are not part of an integrated bariatric surgery program and should serve to decrease complications. However, the need for a light bowel prep for abdominal procedures is questionable.

K. A. Gutowski, MD

Weight Reduction following Abdominoplasty: A Retrospective Case Review Pilot Study

Fuller JC, Nguyen CN, Moulton-Barrett RE (Alameda Hosp, Los Angeles, CA; Univ of California, San Jose; Los Angeles David Geffen School of Medicine, CA; et al)

Plast Reconstr Surg 131:238e-244e, 2013

Background.—The question of whether or not abdominoplasty is associated with permanent weight reduction remains controversial. In coalition, should abdominoplasty be used as an adjunct for weight reduction in the overweight/obese patient?

Methods.—This retrospective patient case series attempts to determine the most important factors associated with weight reduction.

Results.—All patients undergoing abdominoplasty had weight loss beyond that of their resected pannus, with a minimum body mass index reached 11.6 ± 1.7 weeks after surgery. Weight loss is attributed to an increase in satiety by 75 percent ($n = 15$) of patients. Preoperative body mass index greater than or equal to 24.5 kg/m^2 can be used to predict long-term weight loss with a sensitivity and specificity of 92.9 percent and 83.3 percent, respectively. Patients above this threshold achieved significantly more weight loss (−4.5 ± 1.4 percent body mass index) at 1 year compared with their lower body mass index counterparts ($p = 0.014$), as did those with pannus resections weighing greater than 4.5 lb ($p = 0.01$).

Conclusions.—Abdominoplasty performed on patients with a body mass index greater than 24.5 kg/m^2 appears to be linked to sustained weight loss at 1 year. Satiety appears to be a prominent contributing factor, as does the amount of fat resected. Possible neurocrine mechanisms are discussed.

Clinical Question/Level of Evidence.—Therapeutic, IV.

▶ Although this study involved only a small group of patients, it does support what some patients experience after abdominoplasty. Whether the weight loss is caused by neuroendocrine mechanisms, an earlier feeling of satiety (which most patients reported), or lifestyle and dietary changes was not determined. Hopefully, we will see more research in this area along with recommendations for patients who are not successful at weight loss after abdominoplasty.

K. A. Gutowski, MD

"Inverted-Y": A Modified Vest-Over-Pants Abdominoplasty Pattern Following Bariatric Surgery

Bracaglia R, Tambasco D, D'Ettorre M, et al (Catholic Univ of the Sacred Heart, Rome, Italy)

Aesthetic Plast Surg 36:1179-1185, 2012

Background.—The post-bariatric surgery patient presents several challenges to the surgeon. Correction of skin and subcutaneous redundancy can be difficult, particularly in massive-weight-loss patients with horizontal laxity, upper abdominal or flank laxity, and "double-roll" deformities. The aim of our study was to propose our modification of the "vest-over-pants" abdominoplasty technique to exploit all the advantages of the Planas technique in bariatric surgery patients and to solve the problem of extreme epigastric skin redundancy in difficult abdominal contour cases.

Methods.—Sixteen post-bariatric surgery patients (10 females and 6 males, nonsmokers) with moderate to severe epigastric skin laxity were enrolled in the study. They all had undergone a biliopancreatic diversion (BPD) by laparotomy and had undergone this body-contouring procedure from 2006 to 2010.

Results.—After the inverted-Y abdominoplasty, 12 patients (75%) had an uneventful recovery. On the other hand, one subject (6.25%) had a seroma and four (25%) had wound dehiscence and delayed wound healing. No skin necrosis was reported. In one patient (6.25%) scar revision in areas that had delayed healing was performed. The addition of a vertical incision has not led to an increased rate of postoperative complications, but the rates are in line with the satisfactory results described with the Planas technique in bariatric surgery patients. In addition, various advantages have been observed compared to traditional vertical resection patterns.

Conclusion.—This case series has quantitative limitations and further investigations are needed. However, this study suggests that inverted-Y abdominoplasty could be a good compromise between the need to minimize complication rates and ensure an optimum aesthetic result and patient satisfaction rate in some abdominal defects in massive-weight-loss patients.

Level of Evidence IV.—This journal requires that authors assign a level of evidence to each article.

▶ For patients with vertical and horizontal skin excess, as typically seen after significant weight loss, an abdominoplasty with a horizontal incision may not provide as much improvement as with the addition of a vertical incision. This technique is similar to the "fleur de lis" abdominoplasty. Key points are to minimize the lateral undermining (which preserves the perforating blood vessels and decreases wound healing complications) and to do the vertical excision and temporary closure before the horizontal incision. Careful attention should be paid to the length of the lower horizontal incision and to not make the upper horizontal incision too short, which would compromise the aesthetic result.

K. A. Gutowski, MD

How Safe Is Thromboprophylaxis in Abdominoplasty?

Dini GM, Ferreira MCC, Albuquerque LG, et al (Universidade Federal de São Paulo, Brazil)

Plast Reconstr Surg 130:851e-857e, 2012

Background.—Deep vein thrombosis and its most dangerous outcome, pulmonary embolism, are complications with a high incidence in hospitalized patients. In plastic surgery, abdominoplasty is the aesthetic surgery more frequently associated with deep vein thrombosis condition. This study aimed to test the efficacy and safety of oral rivaroxaban for the prevention of venous thromboembolism after abdominoplasty in patients considered to be at risk.

Methods.—In a randomized, double-blind study, 40 patients undergoing abdominoplasty were assigned to receive either oral rivaroxaban (10 mg) or oral placebo once daily for 10 days, beginning 6 to 8 hours after surgery.

Results.—The study was interrupted after 27 operations due to systematic complications. The population operated on was composed of women with a mean age of 38 years. Most patients were Caucasian (85 percent) and had a mean body mass index of 28. The average overall rate of complications was 29.6 percent (large hematomas requiring drainage), and all complications were seen in the study group, with none in the control group.

Conclusions.—Plastic surgery procedures in which large detachment is planned in patients with a moderate risk of deep venous thrombosis should be evaluated with regard to the risk and benefit of thromboembolism prophylaxis. Other measures must be applied and eventually contraindicate a surgical procedure. Further research is needed to complement the data from this work.

▶ Oral rivaroxaban (Xarelto) was approved for deep vein thrombosis (DVT) and pulmonary embolism (PE) prophylaxis for orthopedic surgery in the United States in 2011 and then approved for treatment of DVT and PE in 2012. However, because of the unacceptably high hematoma rate, it does not appear to be useful in abdominoplasty patients (despite abdominal flap to abdominal fascia fixation sutures being used in all cases in this series). Low-molecular-weight heparin may be the better option at this time.

K. A. Gutowski, MD

The impact of the menstrual cycle on intra-operative and postoperative bleeding in abdominoplasty patients

Findikcioglu K, Findikcioglu F, Sezgin B, et al (Gazi Univ Faculty of Medicine Hosp, Ankara, Turkey; TDV 29 Mayis Hosp, Ankara, Turkey; et al)
J Plast Reconstr Aesthet Surg 65:e338-e343, 2012

Background.—Hormonal changes that take place during the menstrual cycle may have an effect on perioperative bleeding. Previous studies have confirmed a relationship between the menstrual cycle and surgical bleeding in rhinoplasty and breast reduction surgery; yet both surgical sites display changes in accordance with sex hormone levels during the menstrual phase.

Aim.—The aim of this study was to determine the effect of the menstrual cycle on perioperative bleeding when undergoing surgeries of sites not directly related to menstrual hormonal changes.

Materials and Methods.—Forty-one patients undergoing abdominoplasty were grouped as group A – perimenstrual (0–7, 21–28 days), group B – periovulatory (8–20 days) and group C – postmenopausal. Intra-operative blood loss was calculated during surgery while postoperative blood loss was determined by measuring the amount of drainage. All menstrual data were recorded. Age, body mass index and weight of the resected tissue were also considered as factors that can affect the amount of bleeding and therefore were also evaluated in terms of significance.

Results.—There was no significant difference between groups regarding intra-operative and postoperative blood loss. Body mass index and weight of the resected tissue had a strong influence on the time of drain removal and the amount of intra-operative and postoperative blood loss.

Conclusion.—This study strongly suggests that the menstrual period does not affect perioperative blood loss for operations on areas less sensitive to sex hormone levels such as the abdomen. In light of the results, we can conclude that the patient's menstrual date is not of vital importance regarding perioperative blood loss when planning surgery for areas with less sensitivity to menstrual hormonal changes.

► The mean blood loss in the 3 groups (perimenstrual, periovulatory, and postmenopausal) was about 350 mL. Lower volumes would be expected if the procedure was done using a tumescent fluid infiltration technique.

K. A. Gutowski, MD

Simple Continuous Suture Versus Continuous Horizontal Mattress Suture for Plication of Abdominal Fascia: Which is Better?

Weissman O, Zmora N, Rozenblatt SM, et al (Sheba Med Ctr, Tel Hashomer, Israel; Tel Aviv Univ, Israel; Hebrew Univ, Jerusalem, Israel)

Aesthetic Plast Surg 36:1015-1018, 2012

Background.—Abdominal fascia plication using a simple continuous suture can sometimes cause tears in the fascia. This problem can be circumvented when the continuous horizontal mattress suture is used. No data exist from comparing the two suturing techniques. The aim of this study was to examine which technique can potentially cause greater tissue damage. The time required to perform each type of suture was also recorded.

Methods.—Wound closure pads were plicated using the simple continuous and continuous horizontal mattress techniques performed by a single operator using Ethilon 2-0 nylon sutures. To verify their resilience, plastic bags were inflated beneath the pads to 30, 60, and 120 mmHg and tears were recorded. The time needed to perform the procedures was recorded using a stopwatch.

Results.—Mean time for the continuous vertical mattress suture was 87 s and for the simple continuous suture 116 s. Tears in the pad that was plicated with the simple continuous pattern were significantly longer than those in the pad plicated with the continuous horizontal mattress pattern (fissure mean length ± SD = 3.958 ± 0.157 vs. 2.736 ± 0.157, respectively, $p < 0.001$). This finding was true for each of the three measured pressures (fissure mean length for 30 mmHg was 3.40 ± 1.807 vs. 2.12 ± 1.709 cm; for 60 mmHg, 3.94 ± 2.90 vs. 2.90 ± 1.893 cm; and for 120 mmHg, 4.54 ± 1.924 vs. 3.19 ± 2.110 cm; $p < 0.001$).

Conclusions.—Continuous horizontal mattress pattern sutures were found to be superior to simple continuous pattern sutures in the suggested model, in terms of suturing time and damage to the pad. Further research in human subjects is still required.

Level of Evidence II.—This journal requires that authors assign a level of evidence to each article. For a full description of these Evidence-Based Medicine ratings, please refer to the Table of Contents or the online Instructions to Authors www.springer.com/00266.

► Horizontal mattress sutures not only save time but also seem to have less pull and tearing in abdominal fascia. Although this study was not done on human tissue, the findings seem to apply. In addition to the horizontal mattress plication sutures, a second suture line (running or interrupted sutures) over the first suture line may reinforce and protect the repair.

K. A. Gutowski, MD

Effectiveness of Wound Closure With V-Loc 90 Sutures in Lipoabdominoplasty Patients

Grigoryants V, Baroni A (Private Practice in Glendale, CA; Kaiser Permanente, Los Angeles, CA)

Aesthet Surg J 33:97-101, 2013

Background.—Barbed sutures have gained wider acceptance, especially among plastic surgeons. However, limited information exists about the effectiveness of wound closure using these sutures.

Objectives.—The authors compare closure times and clinical outcomes of 2-layer wound closure using V-Loc 90 barbed sutures (Covidien, Inc, Mansfield, Massachusetts) with conventional, 3-layer closure with nonbarbed, nonlocking sutures.

Methods.—The lipoabdominoplasty wounds of 30 consecutive patients were divided into 2 equal halves, and the control and study halves of the wound were randomly assigned for each patient. On the control side, a conventional 3-layer wound closure (Scarpa's fascia, deep dermis, and upper dermis) was performed using polyglactin 910 and polyglecaprone 25 sutures. On the study side, the wound was closed in 2 layers (Scarpa's fascia and upper dermis) using a running suture of V-Loc 90 sutures. Closure of each layer and of the entire half of the wound was performed by a single surgeon and timed. Patients were followed for an average of 13 months postoperatively. Postoperative complications were recorded and scar appearance was evaluated with the Vancouver Scar Scale (VSS).

Results.—Data were collected from a total of 30 control and 30 study sides. The mean closure time for each layer was faster with barbed sutures than with nonbarbed sutures, and the total average closure time was 4.4 minutes (36.1%) faster using barbed sutures compared with conventional sutures (7.9 vs 12.3 minutes, respectively; $P < .0001$). Postoperative wound complications occurred in 4 (13.3%) control sides compared with 1 (3.3%) study side of the wound. The VSS scores were similar between the 2 sides. The lateral section of the scar received lower VSS scores than central sections.

Conclusions.—Two-layer wound closure using V-Loc 90 barbed sutures was safe and faster and resulted in fewer postoperative complications than 3-layer closure with conventional, nonbarbed sutures. V-Loc 90 sutures did not produce better scar cosmesis. Wound closure with barbed sutures may be financially and clinically advantageous in lipoabdominoplasty patients as it requires less wound closure time.

▶ Recent studies support the use of bidirectional barbed sutures in body contouring wound closure. The primary measured advantage is decreased wound closure time but at a higher suture cost. This report of unidirectional (V-Loc) sutures showed a modest time savings in closure of abdominoplasty incisions with fewer wound complications compared with nonbarbed sutures. Personal experience with barbed sutures suggests they have better tissue approximation of the superficial facial system and Scarpa's fascia with less pull through, making them the preferred choice for excisional body contouring procedures, particularly in massive weight loss patents with poor tissue strength.

K. A. Gutowski, MD

Use of 2-Octyl Cyanoacrylate Together with a Self-Adhering Mesh (Dermabond™ Prineo™) for Skin Closure Following Abdominoplasty: An Open, Prospective, Controlled, Randomized, Clinical Study

Parvizi D, Friedl H, Schintler MV, et al (Med Univ of Graz, Austria; Univ of Technology Graz, Austria)

Aesthetic Plast Surg 37:529-537, 2013

Background.—Abdominoplasty is one of the most commonly performed procedures in plastic surgery. The appearance of the scar is a major factor that contributes to the aesthetic outcome of the procedure and depends largely on the technique of wound closure. The new Prineo™ wound closure system was introduced to combine the effectiveness of 2-octyl cyanoacrylate (Dermabond™) together with a self-adhering mesh.

Methods.—Fifty-two women and eight men aged between 21 and 65 years who were scheduled for abdominoplasty were included in the study. The total operating times after abdominoplasty of the traditional wound closure technique and the Prineo™-type wound closure technique were compared. Furthermore, an analysis comparing the cost of the two methods was performed. Two weeks after surgery the wounds were examined and graded using the Hollander Cosmesis Scale. At the 6- and 12-month follow-ups, the aesthetic outcome of the abdominal scar was evaluated using the Vancouver Scar Scale. Twelve months after surgery, the patients were asked to answer their part of the Patient Scar Assessment Scale.

Results.—The mean total operating time for the new skin closure system was statistically significantly shorter than that of intradermal sutures. The mean price difference per patient was 104.27€ (134.79$) in favor of Prineo™. The Hollander Cosmesis Scale indicated a significantly more favorable overall result with Prineo™ at 2 weeks after surgery. The Vancouver Scar Scale demonstrated a better cosmetic outcome in favor of Prineo™ 6 and 12 months after surgery. The Patient Scar Assessment Scale scores 12 months after surgery indicated that the patients noted significantly less pain, thickness, and irregularity with Prineo™.

Conclusion.—Based on our results, we conclude that Prineo™ is a safe and effective substitute for superficial skin closure, with good cosmetic results and no increase in wound complications. The use of Prineo™ decreases operative time and cost and enhances the patient's postoperative comfort.

Level of Evidence I.—This journal requires that authors assign a level of evidence to each article. For a full description of these Evidence-Based

Medicine ratings, please refer to the Table of Contents or the online Instructions to Authors www.springer.com/00266.

▶ The Prineo™ wound closure system combines 2-octyl cyanoacrylate (Dermabond™) with a self-adhering mesh strip for the purpose of superficial incision closure. It may be used in place of running subcuticular sutures if deeper sutures allow for skin approximation. Personal experience with Pernio™ on body contouring cases in massive weight loss patients (arms, thighs, abdomens, and breasts) confirms the improved early and late scar appearance. However, the cost of the product (in the United States) was not favorable enough to support its use, especially on cases with many long incisions.

K. A. Gutowski, MD

A New Technique Involving a Spherical Stainless Steel Device to Optimize Positioning of the Umbilicus

Mowlavi A, Huynh PM, Huynh DC, et al (Cosmetic Plastic Surgery Inst, CA; Univ of Cincinnati College of Medicine, OH; Univ of California, Irvine; et al)
Aesthetic Plast Surg 36:1062-1065, 2012

Background.—Creating an aesthetically pleasing umbilicus may be challenging due to various factors that involve the patient limitations and suboptimal techniques available to the surgeon. Although many techniques aim to locate the umbilicus after abdominoplasty, none are ideal. The authors use a new technique involving a stainless steel spherical device for definite location of the new neoumbilicus site.

Methods.—Abdominoplasty with full muscle plication and umbilicoplasty was performed to test the effectiveness of this new technique that involves a stainless steel marble called the Umbilicator. It has a diameter of 1.5 cm and three 2-mm holes drilled 120° apart in an equilateral triangle. The Umbilicator is secured to the inferior and superior dermis of the umbilical stalk to help identify the future location of the umbilicus on the abdominal skin. Once the marble is secured, the superior abdominal flap is redraped and trimmed, the suture is repaired, and the location of the umbilicus is determined by feeling for the smooth spherical surface bump with gentle downward pressure on the overlying abdominal skin located within the proximity of the umbilicus.

Results.—The result of this technique produced a definitive means of identifying and delivering the umbilical stalk during abdominoplasty. This technique has been performed in 23 consecutive abdominoplasty procedures with no difficulties locating the umbilical stalk and no infections resulting from the procedure.

Conclusions.—Accurate identification of the umbilicus provides the ability to create an aesthetically pleasing neoumbilicus, thus optimizing abdominoplasty results.

Level of Evidence IV.—This journal requires that authors assign a level of evidence to each article. For a full description of these Evidence-Based Medicine ratings, please refer to the Table of Contents or the online Instructions to Authors www.springer.com/00266.

▶ This small metal sphere is sutured to the umbilical stalk and then located by palpation over the pulled-down abdominal flap to mark the site for the new umbilical location. The technique seems dependent on the ability to feel the sphere, which may be difficult in thicker abdominal flaps. Perhaps a magnetic locator, as used in localizing integrated tissue expander ports, may be more useful.

K. A. Gutowski, MD

Abdominoplasty Revision Using Tissue Expansion

Kadri OM, Moosa S, Mofid MM (David Geffen School of Medicine at UCLA; San Diego Skin, Inc, La Jolla, CA; Univ of California, San Diego, La Jolla)
Aesthetic Plast Surg 37:538-540, 2013

Postoperative revision after abdominoplasty may be necessary at times to improve contour, remove asymmetries, revise the umbilicus, or improve the scar. This report describes the case of an abdominoplasty performed outside the United States that resulted in an inappropriately high and unattractive scar with an elevated pubic hairline. The patient presented to our clinic 2 years after her initial surgery, and a scar-lowering procedure was performed with the assistance of tissue expansion. The reconstructive effort was staged over a period of 4 months, with an initial procedure to repair several hernias, bury the umbilicus, and place a tissue expander. Over several months, 3.5 L of expansion was performed. During a subsequent surgery, the tissue expander was removed, and the scar was successfully lowered and improved. The healing was uneventful, and the patient was satisfied with the outcome. The final result is exhibited in 1-month follow-up photographs.

Level of Evidence V.—This journal requires that authors assign a level of evidence to each article. For a full description of these Evidence-Based Medicine ratings, please refer to the Table of Contents or the online Instructions to Authors www.springer.com/00266.

▶ High-positioned abdominoplasty scars, whether caused by excessive scar migration or poor initial placement, are uncommon and may be very disappointing to the patient. The use of tissue expansion to recruit upper abdominal tissue to lower the scar placement is an option for patients willing to accept 2 procedures and the associated costs of the expanders.

K. A. Gutowski, MD

Dynamic Definition Mini-Lipoabdominoplasty Combining Multilayer Liposculpture, Fat Grafting, and Muscular Plication

Hoyos AE, Perez ME, Castillo L (Univ of San Martin in Bogota, Colombia; Private Practice, Bogota, Colombia)

Aesthet Surg J 33:545-560, 2013

Background.—There is a select group of women for whom mini-abdominoplasty techniques combined with 3-dimensional liposculpture and fat grafting can effectively correct postpartum deformities.

Objective.—The authors describe a multilayer and 360-degree approach, dynamic definition mini-abdominoplasty (DDM), to create athletic definition and contour and to restore a feminine appearance postpartum.

Methods.—A total of 181 consecutive women ages 20 to 56 years underwent DDM between January 2005 and May 2012. Patients who were a minimum of 6 months postpartum and in good health, with a body mass index below 30, were considered for inclusion in the study. Fat grafting was performed in select cases in the buttocks, deltoids, and/or calves. A satisfaction index (SI) was estimated based on patient survey responses.

Results.—An overall SI of 91.5% was achieved. No major complications were reported. Twenty-nine minor complications included postoperative anemia, seroma, and infection in the surgical wound. In most patients, the postpartum abdomen was restored to an aesthetic and even athletic appearance. Athletic definition to the rectus, arms, trunk, thighs, and buttocks was also achieved. No burns or flap necrosis were reported.

Conclusions.—Dynamic definition mini-abdominoplasty is safe and reproducible. It serves as a viable alternative to a full abdominoplasty in selected cases and for women who wish to restore an athletic and feminine appearance after childbirth.

▶ Few patients are ideal candidates for mini-abdominoplasties, but in those who are, this report details the evolution of the lipoabdominoplasty to the mini-lipoabdominoplasty. Extensive circumferential tuck liposuction with correction of a rectus diastasis using a short incision can yield dramatic results in properly selected patients.

K. A. Gutowski, MD

Dynamic-Definition Male Pectoral Reshaping and Enhancement in Slim, Athletic, Obese, and Gynecomastic Patients Through Selective Fat Removal and Grafting

Hoyos A, Perez M (Universidad de San Martin, Bogota, Colombia; Calle 99 #9A-80 Suite 908, Bogota, Colombia)

Aesthetic Plast Surg 36:1066-1077, 2012

Background.—One of the most appealing characteristics of an athletic male body is a well-defined pectoral area. For decades, implants have been the gold standard method for the treatment of this area, but it is not suitable for every case. The goal was to design a mixed technique combining autologous fat extraction and grafting in an anatomically guided fashion to produce a highly athletic contour in the male pectoral.

Methods.—The patient criteria included a body mass index (BMI) lower than 30 kg/m^2, adequate skin tone, and general good health. A three-phase procedure was performed, beginning with infiltration of tumescent solution and followed by fragmentation of extra fat in an anatomic fashion using internal third-generation ultrasound; extraction that blends deep, intermediate, and superficial fat removal; and multilayer fat grafting in the pectoral area. In the presence of gynecomastia, a selective pull-through technique was used in an anatomic manner.

Results.—In a series of 154 consecutive male patients, the minor complications ($n = 15$) included asymmetries ($n = 10$) and residual gynecomastia ($n = 5$). The major complications ($n = 3$) included unilateral hematoma ($n = 2$), and abscess that required sonographic-guided removal ($n = 1$). An appealing muscular contour was produced in most patients, and the satisfaction rate was very high.

Conclusion.—Implants are no longer the only option for defining and augmenting the male chest. Combining fat grafting in a multilayer fashion with precise anatomic fat and gland removal achieved a contoured and athletic male pectoral in a safe and reproducible manner.

Level of Evidence IV.—This journal requires that authors assign a level of evidence to each article. For a full description of these Evidence-Based Medicine ratings, please refer to the Table of Contents or the online Instructions to Authors www.springer.com/00266.

▶ This article details the advanced aesthetics of the male chest. The procedures involve fat removal, fat repositioning, and fat grafting along with gynecomastia glandular tissue excision. The results are dramatic, but the process requires significant experience and judgment with liposuction. In the right hands, it may offer a better option than pectoral implants for improving the appearance of the male chest.

K. A. Gutowski, MD

Refreshing Labioplasty Techniques for Plastic Surgeons

Triana L, Robledo AM (Clinica Corpus y Rostrum, Cali, Colombia; Universidad del Valle, Cali, Colombia)

Aesthetic Plast Surg 36:1078-1086, 2012

Background.—Patient requests for plastic surgery of the female genitalia have become more common. There are several technical options to manage hypertrophic labia minora, including direct excision, wedge resection, and deepithelialization. Labia majora hypertrophy and hypoplasia can also be managed surgically. The aim of this study was to summarize labioplasty techniques to date, and describe the senior author's technique for labia minora and majora labioplasty.

Methods.—Seventy-four patients underwent direct labia minora excision with or without clitoral hood molding and management of labia majora by the senior author from January 2009 to August 2011.

Results.—The average follow-up time was 6 months. The range of the patients' ages was wide with an average age of 35 years. One patient had an infection and one had wound dehiscence. Six patients had palpable fatty cysts in the labia majora after fat injections; the cysts of five of these patients reabsorbed before 6 months. In one patient a palpable mass persisted 8 months after surgery; however, it was not visible or painful and the patient was satisfied with the result. No cases of scar contracture, painful scar, or discomfort because of labial edge distortion were noted. The satisfaction rate was close to 100 %.

Conclusion.—The direct excision of the excess labia minora is a good technique and does not produce scar-associated problems.

Level of Evidence III.—This journal requires that authors assign a level of evidence to each article.

▶ With the increased awareness of labiaplasty as an aesthetic procedure, concerns have been raised by gynecologists who question the value of the procedure. Although a formal patient-reported outcomes evaluation has not been done, the general opinion is that patients are satisfied with the results. For the plastic surgeon, there are many procedure options but no comparative studies on which is best. Common labia minora procedures are:

- The direct (linear) excision may be simplest and have the fewest healing problems but may result in scar contracture. A modification with a Z- or W-plasty, or a lazy-S incision, may prevent this problem.
- Wedge excisions preserve the normal labia minora edge and color but may also form contracture, and various modifications have been proposed.
- An inferior wedge resection with a superior flap may maintain the normal appearance but is more prone to healing problems.
- A central labial de-epithelialization with direct closure preserves the labial edge but may not be useful for very large labia.

For the labia majora, liposuction, direct excision, and volume replacement (typically with fat grafting) may be done at the same time as the labia minora procedure.

K. A. Gutowski, MD

Aesthetic and Functional Satisfaction After Monsplasty in the Massive Weight Loss Population

Bloom JM, Van Kouwenberg E, Davenport M, et al (Univ of Rochester Med Ctr, NY; et al)

Aesthet Surg J 32:877-885, 2012

Background.—The mons region is often affected by massive weight loss (MWL), with descent of the pubic area and residual adiposity. Thinning and resuspension are often performed concomitantly with abdominal contouring procedures.

Objectives.—Assess patient satisfaction, as well as functional and aesthetic results, after monsplasty in the MWL population.

Methods.—The authors identified 54 consecutive female MWL patients (≥50 lbs) who had undergone abdominal contouring and completed at least 3 months of follow-up as potential subjects. Subjects were asked to complete a Mons Satisfaction Survey, either by phone or in person. Demographic and procedural data were collected from our prospective registry. Descriptive statistics were calculated with significance set at P value < .05.

Results.—Thirty-one patients (57.8%) completed the survey. Average patient age was 46 ± 11.3 years. Mean maximum body mass index (BMI) was 52.0 ± 8.81 kg/m^2, mean current BMI was 31.0 ± 6.22 kg/m^2, and mean delta BMI was 20.7 ± 6.00 kg/m^2. Average pannus resection weight was 3.25 ± 2.03 kg. Visualization of the genitalia improved from 25.8% to 100% (P < .01). Patients rated the appearance of their mons as 3.18 ± 2.11 prior to surgery and 8.58 ± 1.73 after surgery (P < .001) on a scale of 1 to 10. Hygiene improved in 61.3% of patients, and sex life improved in 51.6%, with 32.3% of patients reporting increased genital sensitivity. Incontinence decreased from 22.6% to 12.9%, and 6 patients reported a change in urinary stream.

Conclusions.—Monsplasty at the time of abdominal contouring yields significant improvement in patient satisfaction levels and functional scores. With proper incisional design, monsplasty can be performed safely during abdominal contouring with high patient satisfaction to improve both form and function of the pubic region.

▶ Mons skin and adipose tissue excess and deformity are common in massive weight loss patients but can also be seen in non—weight loss patients presenting for abdominoplasty. Addressing this area during abdominoplasty can provide aesthetic and functional improvement while increasing patient satisfaction. Care should be taken to not thin the mons tissue too much (which may affect the normal padding over the pubic symphysis) or to elevate it too high (which may affect the urinary stream or cause sexual dysfunction).

K. A. Gutowski, MD

Buttock Augmentation with Silicone Implants: A Multicenter Survey Review of 2226 Patients

Mofid MM, Gonzalez R, de la Peña JA, et al (Univ of California San Diego, La Jolla; Univ of Ribeirão Preto, São Paulo, Brazil; Private Practice, Huizquilucan, Mexico; et al)

Plast Reconstr Surg 131:897-901, 2013

Background.—Enhancement of buttock volume with gluteal silicone implants has been performed by surgeons for over 30 years, but no studies have examined complication rates or outcomes of more than single-surgeon experiences. Numerous technical differences in how gluteal augmentation surgery with implants is performed also exist, and to date, surgeon preferences for implant plane, incisional access, implant type, and drain use have not been quantified.

Methods.—A 10-question survey was sent to 83 targeted members of the American Society of Plastic Surgeons requesting information about number of cases performed, duration of surgeon experience, implant placement plane and incisional access, implant type, length of typical surgery, use of drains and antibiotic irrigation solution, surgeon satisfaction and surgeon assessment of patient satisfaction, and number of complications experienced.

Results.—Nineteen respondents (25 percent response rate) provided data on 2226 patients. Thirteen respondents (68.4 percent) favored the intramuscular plane of dissection over the subfascial plane. Preference for incisional access was nearly equally divided between a single incision in the gluteal cleft (10 respondents) and two incisions separated within the cleft (nine respondents). The total number of complications reported was 848 (38.1 percent).

Conclusions.—Gluteal augmentation with silicone implants has gained popularity in the last decade. Despite this, no previous studies have examined multisurgeon experiences with this procedure to determine complication rates or surgeon technical preferences. The authors present data from a survey sent to experienced gluteal augmentation surgeons. Advances in technique and implant options are needed to improve complication rates experienced with this procedure.

► Gluteal implant augmentation has a reputation for high complication rates, but most reports are based on only an individual surgeon's experience. There is a perceived high incidence of infection and a need for implant removal. Although the complication rate in this multicenter analysis appears high, it is not that much different from the core studies of breast augmentation with implants.

Wound dehiscence was the most common complication (8%) in this study (up to 30% in other studies), but the study did not distinguish between superficial spread of the incision and deep wound separation requiring surgical repair. The infection rate in this series was less than 2% for infections requiring implant removal and about 4% for infections that did not require implant removal, which is consistent with past reports. It is possible that infections and wound problems may be higher for surgeons who do not perform buttock augmentation routinely as there are technical aspects of the procedure that can decrease wound and infection complications.

Wound dehiscence can be minimized by a careful, atraumatic technique and by minimizing contamination of the wound. During wound closure, each side of the incision should be tacked down to the presacral fascia to avoid wound tension. The use of multiple layers of absorbable sutures and obliteration of dead space, along with deep dermal sutures, are advocated. Based on personal experience, absorbable, bidirectional barbed sutures are useful in these cases. Use of smaller implants can decrease wound dehiscence by reducing wound tension. Compression shorts and very limited physical activity in the immediate postoperative period are also important.

A limitation of this study is that some of the implants used in this series were not approved (and used) in the United States, so not all the conclusions may apply.

K. A. Gutowski, MD

Calf lipo-reshaping

Hoppmann R, Meruane M, González D, et al (Tabancura Clinic, Santiago, Chile)
J Plast Reconstr Aesthet Surg 66:956-961, 2013

Background.—Augmentation and remodelling of the calf is becoming more and more frequent, representing a challenge for the surgeon who must consider this body zone as a functional and aesthetical whole. Historically, calf reshaping has been carried out with silicone implants, mainly in the subaponeurotic plane; nonetheless, as in other body sites it is possible to perform lipoinjection which is a reliable procedure with minimal scarring and a lasting outcome with rare, long-term complications.

Materials and Methods.—Between the years 2009 and 2011, five patients (three women and two men) underwent bilateral calf liporemodelling. Follow-up was between 6 and 18 months. The larger perimeter of each calf was measured for follow-up.

Magnetic resonance imaging was used to localise the injected fat at the end of the follow-up period in two of the patients.

Results.—An average of 126.8 ± 21.2 cc was lipoinjected into each calf. The average final augmentation in the larger perimeter of each leg was 2.8 cm. All patients obtained a good aesthetical outcome and were satisfied. No important complications were seen in this series.

Conclusion.—According to our experience and outcomes we can recommend the liporemodelling technique of the calf as a valid alternative for the reshaping of the distal third of the inferior extremity.

► Contouring the lower leg is not common, but for patients with a poorly developed calf, augmentation can restore a more balanced appearance. Calf implants are reliable but do have the limitations associated with other prosthetic devices. Augmentation with fat grafting is another option that may allow for more specific contouring. This patient series was small, so more studies are needed. However, based on experience with fat grafting in other body regions, this technique likely plays a major role in outcomes, and additional treatments may be necessary. This may not be an option for body builders and those looking for a more sculpted calf, as the subcutaneous fat injections may not give the appearance of a well-defined muscle. Perhaps subfascial or intramuscular fat placement (about 70% of which was done in this study) may give more natural results.

K. A. Gutowski, MD

1,000 Consecutive Cases of Laser-Assisted Liposuction and Suction-Assisted Lipectomy Managed With Local Anesthesia

Chia CT, Theodorou SJ (128 Central Park South, NY)

Aesthetic Plast Surg 36:795-802, 2012

Background.—Advances in suction-assisted lipectomy (SAL) include improved instrumentation, better understanding of fluid dynamics, and an improved concept of appropriate indications. The tumescent technique uses subcutaneous injection of isotonic fluid containing vasoconstrictive and analgesic agents and is proved to be safe, with low morbidity and mortality rates. Laser-assisted liposuction (LAL) using local infiltration of an anesthetic and no general anesthesia or sedation has been developed, with claims of fat destruction and skin tightening. This study aimed to review 1,000 consecutive cases of LAL and SAL performed with the patient under local anesthesia and to determine whether this represents a safe technique with few complications.

Methods.—During a period of 22 months, 581 consecutive patients (486 females and 95 males) underwent 1,000 LAL/SAL operations, 545 of whom had multiple procedures performed. None of the patients had a body mass index (BMI) higher than 30 kg/m^2. The patients ranged in age from 18 to 62 years. The fat aspirate ranged from 50 to 1,400 ml. Patients were given an oral sedative, an antibiotic, and an analgesic. Ringer's lactate solution containing lidocaine and epinephrine was injected into the subcutaneous space. The 1,064-nm and/or 1,320-nm neodymium: yttrium-aluminum-garnet (Nd:YAG) laser was used for laser lipolysis followed by SAL using standard and/or power-assisted liposuction (PAL) cannulas. The treated areas included the neck, triceps, male breast, midback, flanks, axilla, abdomen, mons pubis, thighs, presacrum, and knees. No patient was administered intravenous sedation or general anesthesia.

Results.—The average number of areas treated was 1.8, and no major complications or mortalities were observed. There were three burns, two infections, one hematoma, and one seroma. A total of 73 secondary procedures were performed (7.3%). No tertiary procedures were required.

Conclusion.—For appropriately selected patients, comparable results can be obtained with an excellent safety profile and short recovery period using LAL and SAL with the patient under local anesthesia. The awake patient is able to participate in body positioning and to provide physiologic monitoring. No major complications occurred in this series. The burn and hematoma complications occurred in the first 25 cases and may have been related to a learning curve. One case of cellulitis occurred in the triceps region, and a second infection occurred in the abdomen. Both responded to antibiotics. Altogether, 73 touch-up procedures (7.3%) were performed. The amounts of fat removal were comparable with the volumes obtained using traditional liposuction. In conclusion, this series demonstrated that LAL/SAL using local anesthesia is a safe procedure for selected patients, with acceptably low morbidity and revision rates.

Level of Evidence IV.—This journal requires that authors assign a level of evidence to each article. For a full description of these Evidence-Based Medicine ratings, please refer to the Table of Contents or the online Instructions to Authors at www.springer.com/00266.

▶ Midface lifts can result in improved facial rejuvenation that cannot always be achieved with a lateral cheek facelift alone. However, the evolution of facial volume replacement with fillers and fat may have resulted in fewer surgical corrections of the midface. The endoscopic approach to the midface helps avoid potential complications involving the lower eyelid but does require a more complex dissection, which puts the temporal branch of the facial nerve at risk (in this series, about half of the patients had a temporary nerve weakness). Another criticism of the endoscopic approach is that it did not always achieve predictable results. Based on long-term follow-up, it now seems that the use of a bioabsorbable fixation system (Endotine) can make the procedure easier with a lower revision rate. Proper patient selection for an isolated midface lift should exclude older patients with facial skin excess who would be better served with a full facelift and those with significant facial volume loss.

K. A. Gutowski, MD

Suction-assisted lipectomy (SAL) for body contouring: infiltration and aspiration ratios revisited

Khan UD (Re-Shape Clinic, Kent, UK)

Eur J Plast Surg 36:359-366, 2013

Background.—With the current advancement in technology, different forms of techniques for liposuction are introduced. However, suction-assisted lipectomy remains the gold standard. Suction-assisted liposuctions can be performed using dry, wet, super-wet, and tumescent techniques based on the use of infiltration volume. A retrospective analysis was carried out to evaluate the outcome of regional body contouring using suction-assisted lipectomy.

Methods.—A retrospective analysis of prospectively collected data of 110 patients who had suction-assisted lipectomy was performed. All patients had their procedure performed by a single surgeon between 2008 and 2009.

Results.—A total of 198 areas were identified in nine regions of 110 patients. Of these patients, 33 were males and 77 females. The mean age of the male patients was 38.2 years (range 19–59, SD ± 9.5), whereas the mean age of the female patients was 41.2 years (range 19–68, SD ± 10.4). The mean body mass index of the patients was 28.6 ± 4.9. The areas included the neck ($n = 19$, inf/asp ratio 1.19), arms ($n = 16$, inf/asp ratio 0.45), chest ($n = 16$, inf/asp ratio 0.75), abdomen ($n = 29$, inf/asp ratio 0.41), inner thigh ($n = 20$, inf/asp ratio 0.49), outer thigh ($n = 30$, inf/asp ratio 0.48), knee (n = 12, inf/asp ratio 0.24), hips ($n = 34$, inf/asp ratio 0.56), and upper back (bra strap area) ($n = 22$, inf/asp ratio 0.65).

Conclusions.—The outcome suggests that body contouring using suction-assisted lipectomy is an effective method when performed using low volume of infiltrate.

Level of Evidence.—Level IV, therapeutic study

▶ Liposuction infiltration solution volume to aspiration volume is commonly between 2 to 1 (super-wet technique) and 3 to 1 (tumescent technique). High infiltration fluid volumes allow for adequate dispersion of local anesthetic, which is not as important in cases done with deep sedation or general anesthesia (as in this series) but is critical when done only using infiltration anesthesia. The vasoconstrictive effects of epinephrine seem to be less dependent on the volume infiltrated. As this study shows, ratios of 0.5 to 1 may be used when performing traditional liposuction under general anesthesia. This, however, may not be true when using enhanced liposuction techniques, such as ultrasound-assisted or laser-assisted liposuction, in which thermal damage may occur if enough fluid is used.

K. A. Gutowski, MD

Liposuction of the Arm Concurrent with Brachioplasty in the Massive Weight Loss Patient: Is It Safe?

Bossert RP, Dreifuss S, Coon D, et al (Univ of Pittsburgh Med Ctr, PA)
Plast Reconstr Surg 131:357-365, 2013

Background.—Brachioplasty continues to be a sought-after procedure among the massive weight loss population. Residual adiposity of the upper arm can make this procedure more difficult. The authors sought to determine the safety of arm liposuction outside the region of excision with concomitant excisional brachioplasty.

Methods.—Data were analyzed from a prospective registry of massive weight loss patients who underwent brachioplasty alone or with concurrent arm liposuction. Variables examined included age, sex, body mass index, method of weight loss, medical comorbidities, and smoking status. Outcomes included complications such as seroma, wound dehiscence, infection, hematoma, lymphedema, and need for revision. Multivariate analyses were performed to assess outcome measures.

Results.—One hundred forty-four patients (139 women and five men; mean body mass index, 29.6 ± 4.1 kg/m^2; mean age, 46 ± 10.7 years) underwent brachioplasty. Sixty-four patients had concomitant arm liposuction at the time of brachioplasty. The remaining 80 patients underwent excisional brachioplasty alone. Despite significantly higher operative body mass indices among those undergoing concurrent liposuction, no significant differences in complication rates were seen between the liposuction and excision-alone cohorts for seroma (19.1 percent versus 23.1 percent), wound dehiscence (7.9 percent versus 2.6 percent), infection (4.8 percent versus 6.4 percent), hematoma (3.2 percent versus 0 percent), or lymphedema (3.2 percent versus 1.3 percent). Revision rates were similar between the two groups (9.5 percent with liposuction and 8.9 percent without liposuction).

Conclusion.—Liposuction can be performed safely and effectively outside the region of excision at the time of brachioplasty without the need for prior debulking or staged arm-contouring procedures.

Clinical Question/Level of Evidence.—Therapeutic, III.

▶ For many patients considering brachioplasty, additional fat debulking with liposuction can give better results. Liposuction followed by brachioplasty as staged procedures is another alternative but requires an additional procedure and may leave the tissue scarred and difficult to contour. Combining the 2 procedures is a reasonable and safe option.

K. A. Gutowski, MD

5 Breast

General

Use of Selective Serotonin Reuptake Inhibitors Antidepressants and Bleeding Risk in Breast Cosmetic Surgery

Basile FV, Basile AR, Basile VV (Basile Med Ctr, Ribeirao Preto, Brazil; Ivo Pitanguy Inst, Botafogo, Brazil)

Aesthetic Plast Surg 37:561-566, 2013

Background.—Selective serotonin reuptake inhibitors (SSRIs) are the most common antidepressant prescribed currently. Data regarding SSRI use among plastic surgery patients may differ between different populations, but the incidence could be as high as 10%. It is known that SSRIs decrease platelet serotonin storage and platelet function, and their association with postsurgical bleeding in mastectomy patients and orthopedic surgery patients is well established. An increased risk of postsurgical bleeding among plastic surgery patients may have important clinical implications, but this has not been evaluated to date. The authors therefore conducted a hospital-based study with prospectively collected data to examine the association between the use of SSRIs and postsurgical bleeding. To the authors' knowledge, this is the first study to evaluate the effects of SSRIs on bleeding risk in the breast cosmetic surgery population.

Methods.—All patients who underwent breast cosmetic plastic surgery procedures (breast augmentation, breast reduction, or mastopexy) at our institution between January of 2001 and December of 2011 were reviewed. The patients were divided into two groups by SSRI use history: a no-use group and an active-use group. The primary end point for a bleeding event was the need for intervention. Patients were further subcategorized by type of breast surgery performed, body mass index, and age. Descriptive statistics tabulated the frequency of a bleeding event within the groups. Logistic regression was applied to evaluate the risk of a bleeding event according to the use of SSRIs. The odds ratios (ORs) with their 95% confidence intervals (CIs) associating SSRI use with postoperative bleeding were computed.

Results.—During the study period, 2,285 patients had breast cosmetic surgery, and 33 of these patients (1.44%) experienced a bleeding event (hematoma requiring surgical draining). Of the 196 patients (8.58%) in the active-use group, 9 (4.59%) experienced a bleeding event. Of the

2,089 patients in the no-use group, 24 (1.15%) presented with bleeding. The patients using SSRIs had a 4.14-fold greater risk of breast hematoma needing intervention than the patients who were not users (OR, 4; 95% CI, 1.90–9.04). Logistic regression also showed that bleeding events were more common among the SSRI users regardless of the type of procedure performed, the body mass index, or the age group.

Conclusions.—Use of SSRIs is associated with a fourfold increased risk of bleeding after breast cosmetic surgery (from 1.44 to 4.59%). The decision of psychologically vulnerable patients to stop SSRIs before surgery should not be made without a complete discussion of the risks and benefits.

Level of Evidence III.—This journal requires that authors assign a level of evidence to each article. For a full description of these Evidence-Based Medicine ratings, please refer to the Table of Contents or the online Instructions to Authors www.springer.com/00266.

▶ The findings in this study are consistent with a large, retrospective medical records review of more than 530 000 patients who underwent surgery at 375 US hospitals between 2006 and 2008, which also found an increased risk of bleeding associated with use of selective serotonin reuptake inhibitors (SSRIs). Although it may be worthwhile to discuss this additional risk with patients, stopping SSRIs before surgery is not yet recommended because of the potential risks of psychiatric alterations. However, for elective cases, the patient and his or her psychiatrist may discuss withholding the SSRI or changing to a different class of antidepressants if possible.

K. A. Gutowski, MD

Does residents' involvement in mastectomy cases increase operative cost? If so, who should bear the cost?

Chamberlain RS, Patil S, Minja EJ, et al (Saint Barnabas Med Ctr, Livingston, NJ; et al)

J Surg Res 178:18-27, 2012

Introduction.—It is a widely held belief that surgical residents' involvement in operative cases increases operative time and costs. However, there is little published data regarding the veracity of this belief, and there is poor documentation of the actual costs associated with involving surgical residents in operative cases. This report represents a retrospective analysis of the additional cost associated with involving surgical residents of all training years in mastectomy cases over a 6-y period.

Methods.—A total of 1063 mastectomy cases (with and without reconstruction) were performed over a 6-y period (2004–2010) at the Saint Barnabas Medical Center, Livingston, NJ. Data relating to the type of mastectomy performed, operative times, training level of residents involved, and the surgical attendings' case volume were collected. Two major groups (attendings-only and attendings with residents) and 19 mastectomy subcategories were formed. Differences in operating room (OR) times between the attendings-only and attendings with residents groups were multiplied by the hospital OR charges per minute of time ($15/min after the initial 30 min) to determine the additional operative costs associated with residents' involvement. The impact of postgraduate training year and the attendings' case volume on operative time was analyzed separately. Statistical analysis was conducted using IBM SPSS 18.0.1 Windows version (PASW Statistics for Windows, SPSS Inc, Chicago).

Results.—Twenty-six surgeons and 97 residents were involved in 1063 mastectomy cases. Eight hundred ninety-five cases involved residents, of which 405 cases had reconstruction and 490 cases did not. Among 168 cases involving residents, 107 cases had reconstruction and 61 cases did not. The mean OR time was increased in nearly all cases involving surgical residents but statistically significant in only nine of the 19 mastectomy subcategories. Postgraduate year (PGY) 1 or PGY2 residents increased OR time for unilateral mastectomy, whereas the involvement of PGY1 through PGY3 residents increased OR time for bilateral mastectomy + reconstruction ($P < 0.05$). No significant difference was observed when PGY4 and PGY5 were involved in mastectomy cases. The additional calculated time required to perform mastectomies involving surgical residents was 41,366 min, which corresponded to an increase in OR costs of $620,340 over 6 y.

Conclusion.—The involvement of surgical residents in mastectomy cases significantly increases operative times and cost. This difference is most apparent when junior-level residents are involved and disappears by the PGY4–PGY5. Increased operative costs and the lost opportunity costs for surgical attendings are significant issues associated with residency education. Center for Medicare and Medicaid Services and Accreditation Council on Graduate Medical Education should consider such data when establishing appropriate reimbursements for graduate training programs.

▶ Medical education is an expensive proposition for those involved in receiving and providing it as well as for society, which directly and indirectly benefits from it. The authors are to be commended for undertaking this study and more need to be performed if we are to bring clarity and understanding to the true net "costs" of medical education as opposed to merely looking at the gross costs of education (eg, as increased costs associated with increased operative times vs service benefits that accrue from resident care provided). Not surprisingly, involvement of residents, primarily junior ones, results in increased operative time as compared with surgery performed by staff surgeons only and also those cases in which senior residents (postgraduate years 4 and 5) participated. The large number of subcategories makes these data a bit difficult to assess. Data reflecting mastectomy and reconstruction, by the authors own admission, are less reliable because of the difficulty in separating times for mastectomy alone, performed by staff and residents, from reconstruction performed primarily by staff surgeons. One of the major challenges for the future of surgical education and curriculum will be to maximize the acquisition of knowledge and skills in a climate of simulation and virtual reality before the residents come to the operating room.[1]

S. H. Miller, MD

Reference

1. Haluck RS, Krummel TM. Computers and virtual reality for surgical education in the 21st century. *Arch Surg*. 2000;135:786-792.

Augmentation and Silicone

Secondary Augmentation Mammaplasties and Periprosthetic Infection: A Three-Year Retrospective Review

Khan UD (Private Practice in London, UK)
Aesthet Surg J 32:465-473, 2012

Background.—Secondary or revision surgery following primary augmentation mammaplasty is common. There are several published studies on the incidence and prevention of infection after primary augmentation mammaplasty, but there is a paucity of information on the incidence of periprosthetic infection after secondary or revision augmentation mammaplasty procedures.

Objectives.—The author evaluates the incidence of periprosthetic infection in a series of revision and secondary mammaplasty patients from his practice.

Methods.—A retrospective review was performed of the charts for 92 consecutive patients who underwent bilateral secondary mammaplasty with the author between July 2008 and April 2011. Each breast was taken as a single unit, for a total of 184 breasts. The data were compiled and compared with previous studies related to periprosthetic infection following primary augmentation mammaplasty.

Results.—The average age of the patients was 35.8 ± 7.9 years (range, 19-54 years). One patient developed unilateral periprosthetic infection in her left breast. This incidence of 0.54% was comparable to infection incidence of 0.5% for primary augmentation mammaplasty previously reported by the author.

Conclusions.—In this series, there was no higher incidence of infection seen in secondary augmentation mammaplasty than was seen in previous studies on primary mammaplasty.

Level of Evidence.—4.

▶ This is an interesting article of one surgeon's experience. I am not sure what can be generalized from this study, as it is retrospective and has a very small outcome: 1 postoperative breast infection in the secondary group for an incidence (0.54%) equivalent to that of infection in his primary augmentation patients. Most interesting is the failure of swab cultures of the capsules to identify bacteria. Would more information have been gleaned by culturing surgical capsular specimens? Other issues that still need clarification are the benefits and risks of using povidone iodine as an irrigation solution and the prolonged 5-day use of oral prophylactic antibiotics after the initial single intravenous dose of cephalosporin. It would seem to me that one of the plastic surgical organizations in this country should be capable of issuing best practice guidelines for local antibacterial therapy and systemic antibiotics in breast augmentation, both primary and secondary.

S. H. Miller, MD

Cancer and Reconstruction

Total Skin-Sparing Mastectomy: A Systematic Review of Oncologic Outcomes and Postoperative Complications

Piper M, Peled AW, Foster RD, et al (Univ of California, San Francisco)
Ann Plast Surg 70:435-437, 2013

Introduction.—Despite the potential aesthetic and psychological benefits of total skin-sparing mastectomy (TSSM) with preservation of the nipple-areolar complex (NAC) skin, there is still reluctance to use the technique due to concern for increased recurrence rates or higher postoperative complication rates. The rapidly expanding literature describing outcomes after TSSM enables a comprehensive review of recurrence rates and surgical complications.

Methods.—Studies describing nipple-sparing or TSSM were identified from the MEDLINE and Cochrane databases. Studies that reported oncologic outcomes and/or data on postoperative complications were included.

Results.—Twenty-seven studies were identified that met inclusion criteria, representing a total of 3331 mastectomies. Review of oncologic outcomes in the 10 studies (representing 1148 mastectomies) with documented mean/median follow-up of 2 years demonstrated an overall local-regional recurrence rate of 2.8%. Ischemic complications involving the NAC were reported in 24 studies (representing 3091 mastectomies), with 9.1% of cases reported to have some degree of NAC necrosis and 2.0% of cases complicated by complete necrosis leading to NAC loss. Sixteen studies (representing 2213 mastectomies) reported rates of skin flap necrosis, which occurred in 9.5% of cases. Eighty-one percent of the total cases reviewed involved expander-implant reconstruction; in the 16 studies (representing 2343 reconstructions) that reported outcomes after expander-implant reconstruction, overall expander-implant loss was 3.4%.

Conclusions.—There is now a significant body of literature demonstrating low rates of early local-regional recurrence and postoperative complications after TSSM. These data support the use of TSSM techniques, which improve psychological and aesthetic outcomes without compromising therapeutic efficacy.

▶ Overall, the results of this study are quite heartening. There is little question in my mind, at least based on many anecdotal reports and intuition, that the aesthetic and psychological outcomes after total skin-sparing mastectomy with preservation of the nipple areolar complex (NAC) are better than the results achieved with total breast and NAC reconstruction. Concerns for safety from an oncologic standpoint are encouraging; however, after reading this study, longer-term follow-up is mandatory, as in those studies in which patients were followed up for more than 5 years, local recurrence almost doubled from 2.7% to 4.4%. The authors also correctly make note of an ever-increasing body of evidence that complications, such as skin-flap necrosis, NAC necrosis, and expander-implant loss, are less likely in institutions or practices with high volumes.

S. H. Miller, MD

A Paradigm Shift in U.S. Breast Reconstruction: Increasing Implant Rates

Albornoz CR, Bach PB, Mehrara BJ, et al (Memorial Sloan-Kettering Cancer Ctr, NY)

Plast Reconstr Surg 131:15-23, 2013

Background.—Despite its benefits in body image, self-esteem, sexuality, and quality of life, historically fewer than 25 percent of patients undergo immediate breast reconstruction. After passage of the Women Health and Cancer Rights Act, studies failed to demonstrate changes in reconstructive rates. A recent single-year report suggests significant shifts in U.S. breast reconstruction patterns. The authors' goal was to assess long-term trends in rates and types of immediate reconstruction.

Methods.—A serial cross-sectional study of immediate breast reconstruction trends was performed using the Nationwide Inpatient Sample database from 1998 to 2008. Data on mastectomies, reconstructive method (autologous/implant), and sociodemographic/hospital predictors were obtained.

Results.—Immediate breast reconstruction rates increased on average 5 percent per year, from 20.8 percent to 37.8 percent ($p < 0.01$). Autologous reconstruction rates were unchanged. Implant use increased by an average of 11 percent per year ($p < 0.01$), surpassing autologous methods as the leading reconstructive modality after 2002. The strongest predictors of implant use were procedures performed after 2002, bilateral mastectomies, patients operated on in Midwest/West regions, and Medicare recipients. In contrast to bilateral mastectomies, which increased by 17 percent per year ($p < 0.01$), unilateral mastectomies decreased by 2 percent per year ($p < 0.01$). Bilateral mastectomy defects had significantly higher reconstruction rates than unilateral counterparts ($p < 0.01$).

Conclusions.—The significant rise in immediate reconstruction rates in the United States correlates closely to a 203 percent expansion in implant use. Although the reason for the increase in implant use is multifactorial, changes in mastectomy patterns, such as increased use of bilateral mastectomies, are one important contributor.

▶ Although these authors expend a great deal of time discussing and analyzing the paradigm shift favoring implant reconstructions of the breast after mastectomy, the reasons for the shift appear to be multifactorial, some readily explainable and others needing more intensive focus. However, what seems to be important about this study is its longitudinal nature, which allows for analysis of trends, especially the apparent association between passage of the Women's Health and Cancer Rights Act and a significantly increased rate of immediate breast reconstruction after mastectomy. The reasons for the increased incidence for the use of implants for breast reconstruction seems intuitive for several groups: patients undergoing bilateral mastectomies (many removing the contralateral breast for prophylaxis), the decreased morbidity for initial reconstruction using implants vs autologous tissue reconstruction, the preference of the physician performing the reconstruction, and the increased confidence in silicone implants, at least for the moment. It is important to continue to follow these trends and to document and share them with colleagues on a regular basis. Of course, several areas unexplored in this study include whether these trends favoring implant reconstructions are altered when examining delayed reconstructions and whether mastectomy and immediate reconstruction is or will be performed on an outpatient basis, as the latter would not be captured in the inpatient sample database.

S. H. Miller, MD

How patients evaluate breast reconstruction after mastectomy, and why their evaluation often differs from that of their clinicians

Beesley H, Ullmer H, Holcombe C, et al (Royal Liverpool Univ Hosp, England, UK; et al)

J Plast Reconstr Aesthet Surg 65:1064-1071, 2012

Introduction.—The evaluation of breast reconstruction after treatment for cancer sometimes differs between the patient who receives it and the surgeon who performs it. Questionnaire studies shed little light on this. We therefore aimed to discover what factors influence how patients evaluate breast reconstruction and thereby to understand sources of disagreement between practitioners and patients in their evaluation.

Methods.—At the study centre, patients who undergo reconstruction following breast cancer rate their subjective evaluation of the procedure, and the surgeon and breast care nurse jointly rate their assessment of cosmesis. We interviewed in depth 27 patients with a range of scores on each rating to elicit the reasons for their evaluations. Interviews were analysed qualitatively with particular attention to patients whose evaluations diverged from those of practitioners.

Results.—Influences on patients' subjective evaluations included two aspects of cosmesis (how 'normal' they felt and how normal or attractive they thought they appeared to others), but also how much they trusted and respected their practitioners and felt cared for by them, whether reconstruction had helped to complete their 'cancer journey' and post-operative complications.

Conclusion.—Patients' subjective evaluation of reconstruction after cancer treatment extends well beyond cosmesis, and experience of cancer influences what they consider important. Evaluations therefore often differ from those of practitioners. Surgeons and specialist nurses need to be aware of the factors that influence patients' evaluations in order to guide patients appropriately in decisions about surgery, and to evaluate outcomes across the domains that matter to patients.

▶ This is a very important topic that all plastic surgeons performing breast reconstruction need be aware of. For years, reports of postoperative results after reconstruction just took into account the perceptions of the surgeon, the surgeon's staff, or colleagues. More recently, reports also began to assess the perceptions of patients regarding satisfaction levels after breast reconstruction using patient satisfaction surveys. The conundrum is often that the professional assessment did not agree with that of the patient's assessment. The issue as identified by these authors reflects that patient assessment of the success of reconstruction goes far beyond the question of satisfaction with the cosmetic result, the primary concern of health professionals, but includes the context and totality of the entire cancer treatment experience. One of the major factors, not surprisingly, is the relationship of the surgeon and the patient—specifically trust in the surgeon. This is really a variant of well-known phenomenon called the "Halo Effect," originally described by Edward Thorndike in 1920.[1] The key take-away message is that although quality control mandates that we improve our outcomes, not all of the patients' expectations can be met and not all of the disappointments are under the control of the surgeon. This is a study from a single institution, and less than 1/3 of the patients available for study actually participated. Further research in this area would certainly be worthwhile.

S. H. Miller, MD

Reference

1. Thorndike EL. A Constant error in psychological ratings. *J Appl Psychol.* 1920;4: 25-29.

Patterns of Use and Patient Satisfaction with Breast Reconstruction among Obese Patients: Results from a Population-Based Study

Kulkarni AR, Katz S, Hamilton AS, et al (Univ of Michigan Med Ctr, Ann Arbor; Univ of Southern California, Los Angeles, CA; Cancer Inst of New Jersey, New Brunswick)

Plast Reconstr Surg 130:263-270, 2012

Background.—The national obesity epidemic is contributing to an increased proportion of overweight and obese breast cancer patients. The authors' purpose was to determine whether patterns of use and outcomes of reconstruction differed among obese and nonobese patients.

Methods.—The authors performed a 5-year follow-up survey of mastectomy-treated breast cancer patients from the Los Angeles and Detroit Surveillance, Epidemiology and End Results Cancer Registries (response rate, 59 percent). Patients were divided into three body mass index categories: normal weight (body mass index <25 kg/m^2), overweight (25 to 30 kg/m^2), and obese (>30 kg/m^2). Outcomes of interest were receipt of reconstruction, type and timing of reconstruction, access barriers, and satisfaction. Chi-square and *t* tests were used for analysis. Logistic regression was used to identify predictors of autologous reconstruction.

Results.—Of 374 mastectomy-treated patients, receipt of reconstruction did not vary by body mass index (53 percent normal weight, 48 percent overweight, and 45 percent obese; $p = 0.43$). Receipt did vary by type of reconstruction: significantly more obese patients received transverse rectus abdominis musculocutaneous flaps compared with normal weight patients (53 percent versus 26 percent; $p = 0.01$). No specific access barriers to reconstruction were identified. Patient satisfaction with surgical decision-making and surgical outcomes was similar across body mass index categories.

Conclusions.—Obese compared with normal weight breast cancer patients have similar use of breast reconstruction, are more likely to receive an autologous procedure, and report similar satisfaction with surgical outcomes. Future efforts should be directed at decreasing the surgical risk in this challenging patient population.

Clinical Question/Level of Evidence.—Therapeutic, II.

▶ This is an interesting article, as it looks specifically at the issue of the likelihood of breast reconstruction in obese patients in the Detroit and Los Angeles areas based on data from their respective Surveillance, Epidemiology and End Results Cancer Registries, not institutional data. It is gratifying to discover that obese patients are being given opportunities to undergo breast reconstruction and that they are generally as well satisfied with outcomes as nonobese patients. It is of interest that the authors focus on the lack of concern for surgical complications in their obese patient population, when, in fact, it was no different than that in the other 2 categories of patients. However, what was different was that the obese patients required more help in trying to lose weight preoperatively than did the overweight and normal-weight patients, an issue not confined to surgical patients by any means. Finally, this study is a bit skewed to those patients in a higher socioeconomic strata.

S. H. Miller, MD

Randomized clinical trial on the effect of fibrin sealant on latissimus dorsi donor-site seroma formation after breast reconstruction

Llewellyn-Bennett R, Greenwood R, Benson JR, et al (Univ of Bristol and Univ Hosps of Bristol NHS Foundation Trust, UK; Addenbrooke's Hosp NHS Foundation Trust, Cambridge, UK)

Br J Surg 99:1381-1388, 2012

Background.—Latissimus dorsi (LD) flap procedures comprise 50 per cent of breast reconstructions in the UK. They are frequently complicated by seroma formation. Fibrin sealants may reduce seroma volumes at the donor site. The aim was to investigate the effect of fibrin sealant (Tisseel®) on total seroma volumes from the breast, axilla and back (donor site) after LD breast reconstruction. Secondary outcomes were specific back seroma volumes together with incidence and severity of wound complications.

Methods.—Consecutive women undergoing implant-assisted or extended autologous LD flap reconstruction were randomized to either standard care or application of fibrin sealant to the donor-site chest wall. All participants were blinded for the study duration but assessors were only partially blinded. Non-parametric methods were used for analysis.

Results.—A total of 107 women were included (sealant 54, control 53). Overall back seroma volumes were high, with no significant differences between control and sealant groups over 3 months. Fibrin sealant failed to reduce *in situ* back drainage volumes in the 10 days after surgery, and did not affect the rate or volume of seromas following drain removal.

Conclusion.—This randomized study, which was powered for size effect, failed to show any benefit from fibrin sealant in minimizing back seromas after LD procedures.

▶ This is an important study for all surgeons performing postmastectomy breast reconstruction with latissimus dorsi flaps (LD) to carefully review. The authors were unable to detect any statistically significant difference between the controls and treated groups using a slow-acting fibrin sealant, Tisseel. Of note is that the authors recorded not only drainage from the back, but also from the mastectomy site and axilla, because they suggest that seromas developing after LD flaps may have contributions from both the mastectomy and axillary sites. The participants recording the outcomes were nurses who were blinded as to whether the patients were treated with the tissue sealant or not; the surgeons were not blinded. Although no significant differences were recorded in this study compared with other studies,[1,2] one must be aware that these authors recorded seroma formation from sites other than just the back. Furthermore, the patients treated with sealant did trend to having 20% less overall fluid, drains plus seroma, than the untreated group. Would more patients, higher power than the authors chose, have made this a significant finding? Would another sealant, one that set more rapidly, have given different results? Would quilting at the mastectomy and axillary site have reduced the overall fluid accumulation?

S. H. Miller, MD

References

1. Daltrey I, Thomson H, Hussien M, Krishna K, Royter Z, Winters ZE. Randomized clinical trials of the effects quilting latissimus dorsi flap donor site on seroma formation. *Br J Surg*. 2006;93:825-830.
2. Carless PA, Henry DA. Systemic review and meta-analysis of the use of fibrin sealant to prevent seroma formation after breast cancer surgery. *Br J Surg*. 2006;93:810-819.

Comparison of Sterile Versus Nonsterile Acellular Dermal Matrices for Breast Reconstruction

Buseman J, Wong L, Kemper P, et al (Univ of Kentucky, Lexington)

Ann Plast Surg 70:497-499, 2013

Background.—Acellular dermal matrix (ADM) has been associated with an increased incidence of complications after implant-based breast reconstruction. Recently, sterile ADM has been introduced in an attempt to minimize these complications. To analyze the impact of this product on patient outcomes, we created a database of patients undergoing implant-based breast reconstruction.

Methods.—Patients undergoing implant-based breast reconstruction at the University of Kentucky Medical Center from January 1, 2011, to December 31, 2011 were identified. A database of patient characteristics and outcomes was created. Outcomes investigated included mastectomy flap necrosis, dehiscence, infection, red breast, capsular contracture, hematoma, and seroma. Statistical analysis was performed.

Results.—Fifty-eight patients underwent breast reconstruction with implants or tissue expanders. Of the 58 patients, 9 had the sterile form of ADM placed, 25 had the original aseptic but not sterile ADM, and 24 were not reconstructed with ADM. The most frequent complication noted was seroma, occurring in 6/9 patients with sterile ADM as compared to 2/25 with the aseptic ADM. This was statistically significant ($P = 0.003$).

Conclusions.—The use of sterile ADM is associated with a statistically significant increase in seroma formation. The etiology of this increased incidence remains unknown, but it correlates with the introduction of the sterile form of ADM at our institution. A different preparation or sterilization process, or some other variable as yet unknown, may be responsible. Further studies comparing the different forms of ADM in an animal model may serve to clarify this issue.

► The topic of acellular dermal matrix (ADM) and breast reconstruction has been used and discussed in the plastic surgical literature for almost 9 years, yet the complete story of all of its benefits and risks are undefined. For some reason, virtually all of the reports to date are retrospective and poorly, if at all, controlled. Clearly, this is an area for one or several of the major plastic surgical organizations to develop a multi-institutional, prospective, controlled study looking at the different brands of ADM, both in sterile and nonsterile versions, including the methods or substances for sterilization, to determine whether the risks of infection and seroma justify its continued use and under what circumstances. To date, it is obvious that the current studies seem to document a higher incidence of both infection and seroma with the use of acellular dermal matrix in breast reconstruction.

S. H. Miller, MD

Postoperative Antibiotic Prophylaxis for Implant-Based Breast Reconstruction with Acellular Dermal Matrix

Avashia YJ, Mohan R, Berhane C, et al (Univ of Miami Miller School of Medicine, FL; Johns Hopkins Univ, Baltimore, MD)

Plast Reconstr Surg 131:453-461, 2013

Background.—The use of acellular dermal matrix in implant-based breast reconstruction has been described for improving inferolateral prosthesis coverage and support and inframammary fold reconstruction. Recommended guidelines for infection prophylaxis are the same as for any clean procedure—antibiotic administration only before surgery. Previous studies have demonstrated increased postoperative rates of infection and seroma associated with the use of acellular dermal matrix. The authors evaluated the impact of postoperative antibiotic prophylaxis on infection rates in postmastectomy expander-based breast reconstruction with acellular dermal matrix.

Methods.—A retrospective study reviewed data of 96 patients who underwent either immediate or delayed expander-based breast reconstruction using AlloDerm allogenic acellular dermal matrix. Infection rates were analyzed after patients received postoperative antibiotic prophylaxis for at least 48 hours compared with those who received only perioperative antibiotics.

Results.—Infection rates for breast reconstructions with a postoperative antibiotic course were 7.9 and 3.2 percent. Patients with only perioperative antibiotics had an infection rate of 31.6 percent. Infections were defined by the endpoint of implant removal. Patient demographics, comorbidities, and intraoperative variables were recorded. Uncontrolled variables were time course between mastectomy and reconstruction, nodal dissection, operative history, and whether reconstruction was unilateral or bilateral.

Conclusions.—This study demonstrates significant differences in the rate of infection between the groups of patients undergoing the first stage of two-stage implant-based breast reconstruction who received postoperative antibiotic prophylaxis and the group that received only perioperative antibiotics. This study suggests that the optimal duration of postoperative antibiotic prophylaxis is at least 48 hours (Table 2).

▶ Does 48 hours of antibiotic prophylactic reduce the incidence of postoperative infection in postmastectomy expander breast reconstruction using both tissue expanders and acellular dermis? In this small, retrospective study, the authors suggest that it does when compared with a group of patients in whom only perioperative antibiotics were given. Frankly, after reading this article, I remain unconvinced and believe the premise is sufficiently important to necessitate a multi-institutional, prospective, double-blind study with clearly defined guidelines and parameters involving the use of antibiotics, drains, and diagnosis of infection and seroma. Furthermore, it would be useful to break out immediate and delayed reconstructions in light of some of the suggestions that the second stage of the reconstruction, placement of the final implant, only

TABLE 2.—Patient Demographics, Patient-Specific Risk Factors, and Intraoperative Variables

Characteristics	≤24 Hr Perioperative Antibiotics Only (%)	≥48 Hr Postoperative Antibiotics First Time Interval (%)	≥48 Hr Postoperative Antibiotics Second Time Interval (%)	Statistical Comparison (p)*
Infection rate ($n = 138$)	6/19 (31.6)	7/88 (7.9)	1/31 (3.2)	0.002†
Age, yr	51.2	50.3	52.2	0.97
BMI, m^2/kg	26	27	25.6	0.92
Diabetes	0/19 (0)	10/88 (11.4)	0/31 (0)	0.59
Tobacco use	2/19 (10.5)	19/88 (21.6)	14/31 (45.2)	0.68
Hypertension	1/19 (5.3)	18/88 (20.5)	3/31 (9.7)	0.28
Previous irradiation	2/19 (10.5)	6/88 (6.8)	3/31 (9.7)	1
Previous chemotherapy	3/19 (15.8)	27/88 (30.7)	5/31 (16.1)	0.73
Bilateral reconstruction	7/19 (36.8)	23/88 (16.1)	12/31 (38.7)	0.36
Delayed reconstruction	2/19 (10.5)	17/88 (19.3)	4/31 (12.9)	0.72
Axillary lymph node dissection	11/19 (57)	22/88 (25.0)	12/31 (38.7)	0.27
Tissue expander size, ml	413.2	403.7	326.7	0.25
Intraoperative TE fill volume, ml	232.6	162.8	175.6	0.01
Removal of JP drain 1, POD	8.8	9.58	8.1	0.19
Removal of JP drain 2, POD	16.72	20.68	16.65	0.23

BMI, body mass index; TE, tissue expander; JP, Jackson-Pratt; POD, postoperative day.
*Groups administered antibiotics for 48 hr or longer were combined when compared with the group administered perioperative antibiotics.
†$p > 0.05$ (statistically significant).

requires perioperative antibiotics because "of vascular delay of the flaps and time for integration of the acellular dermis." Clearly this needs further study. Finally, it should be mentioned that in the group receiving perioperative antibiotics only, the fill volume of the tissue expander was significantly greater than in either of the experimental groups receiving postoperative antibiotics (Table 2).

S. H. Miller, MD

Once Is Not Enough: Withholding Postoperative Prophylactic Antibiotics in Prosthetic Breast Reconstruction Is Associated with an Increased Risk of Infection

Clayton JL, Bazakas A, Lee CN, et al (Univ of North Carolina at Chapel Hill)
Plast Reconstr Surg 130:495-502, 2012

Background.—There has been a trend toward limiting perioperative prophylactic antibiotics, based on research not conducted in plastic surgery patients. The authors' university hospital instituted antibiotic prescribing guidelines based on the Surgical Care Improvement Project. An increased rate of surgical-site infections was noted in breast reconstruction patients.

The authors sought to determine whether the change in antibiotic prophylaxis regimen affected rates of surgical-site infections.

Methods.—A retrospective study compared patients undergoing breast reconstruction who received preoperative and postoperative prophylactic antibiotics with a group who received only a single dose of preoperative antibiotic. Type of reconstruction and known risk factors for implant infection were noted.

Results.—Two hundred fifty patients were included: 116 in the pre–Surgical Care Improvement Project group and 134 in the Surgical Care Improvement Project group. The overall rate of surgical-site infections increased from 18.1 percent to 34.3 percent ($p = 0.004$). Infections requiring reoperation increased from 4.3 percent to 16.4 percent ($p = 0.002$). Multivariate logistic regression demonstrated that patients in the Surgical Care Improvement group were 4.74 times more likely to develop a surgical-site infection requiring reoperation (95 percent CI, 1.69 to 13.80). Obesity, history of radiation therapy, and reconstruction with tissue expanders were associated with increased rates of surgical-site infection requiring reoperation.

Conclusions.—Withholding postoperative prophylactic antibiotics in prosthetic breast reconstruction is associated with an increased risk of surgical-site infection, reoperation, and thus reconstructive failure. The optimal duration of postoperative prophylactic antibiotic use is the subject of future study.

Clinical Question/Level of Evidence.—Therapeutic, III.

▶ The authors propose that the antibiotic regimen proposed in the Surgical Care Improvement Project (SCIP) is flawed as it relates to surgical infections rates in breast reconstruction in their institution. At the outset, it appears that they have demonstrated, at least statistically, their hypothesis, but closer reading reveals several flaws. The authors state that they used a stricter definition of infection than exists in the plastic surgery literature, but one wonders why, if they were adhering to the Guideline for Prevention of Surgical Site Infections, 1999,[1] they did not just use the Guidelines criteria for surgical site infection. Additionally, because the SCIP allows one or more postoperative antibiotic dosages within 24 hours of the conclusion of the procedure, why did they arbitrarily choose not to so? Finally, the 2 groups, studied at 2 different time periods, were not similar with regard to obesity, radiation therapy, and chemotherapy rates, but perhaps not statistically demonstrable. The authors, if they wish to challenge the Guidelines proposed, need to perform a more tightly controlled and randomized study, blinded if possible, using the precise criteria and protocols developed by the SCIP.

S. H. Miller, MD

Reference

1. Mangram AJ, Horan TC, Pearson ML, Silver LC, Jarvis WR. Guideline for prevention of surgical site infection, 1999. Hospital Infection Control Practices Advisory Committee. *Infect Control Hosp Epidemiol.* 1999;20:250-280.

Improving outcomes in microsurgical breast reconstruction: Lessons learnt from 406 consecutive DIEP/TRAM flaps performed by a single surgeon

Damen THC, Morritt AN, Zhong T, et al (Erasmus Univ Med Centre, Rotterdam, The Netherlands; Univ Health Network, Toronto, Ontario, Canada)

J Plast Reconstr Aesthet Surg 66:1032-1038, 2013

Background.—Multiple preoperative, intraoperative and postoperative decisions can influence the outcome of microsurgical breast reconstruction. We have simplified the decision-making process by incorporating a number of algorithms into our microsurgical breast reconstruction practice and critically review our results in this study.

Methods.—Prospectively maintained databases for all microsurgical breast reconstructions performed by a single surgeon over a nine-year period were examined to determine: patient demographics; operative details including flap choice, donor and recipient vessel selection; and, details of intraoperative and early postoperative (<six weeks) complications and their management.

Results.—406 Consecutive free flap microsurgical breast reconstructions (164 unilateral and 121 bilateral) were performed in 285 patients over the study period. Deep inferior epigastric artery perforator (DIEP) flaps (88%, $n = 359$) were used most commonly followed by muscle-sparing transverse rectus abdominis musculocutaneous (MS-TRAM) flaps (11%, $n = 44$), and fascial-sparing TRAM (FS-TRAM) flaps (0.7%, $n = 3$). One-hundred-seventy-one (48%) DIEP flaps were based on a single perforator while 188 (52%) had multiple perforators. The internal mammary (IM) artery and vein were used as the recipient vessels for 99% ($n = 403$) of flaps. A second venous anastomosis was required for 11.8 percent ($n = 48$) of flaps. Partial flap failure occurred in nine (2.2%) flaps while total flap failure occurred in two flaps (0.5%). Minimum follow-up was three months.

Conclusions.—Incorporating a number of algorithms into our practice has enabled us to simplify the decision-making processes involved in microsurgical breast reconstruction and to consistently obtain successful surgical outcomes.

▶ This group previously reported on their early series of 175 deep inferior epigastric artery perforator flap reconstructions showing that a learning curve of approximately 30 flaps was necessary to acquire sufficient experience for surgical complication rates to plateau. Now the group presents 406 consecutive free-flap microsurgical breast reconstructions. They have developed algorithms for flap selection, the management of venous congestion, and partial flap necrosis. These have helped simplify decision making and achieve successful surgical outcomes. This is a well thought out, complete, and critical analysis. There is much to be learned from their experience.

D. J. Smith, Jr, MD

6 Grafts, Flaps, and Microsurgery

Grafts

Skin Grafts Provide Durable End-bearing Coverage for Lower-extremity Amputations With Critical Soft Tissue Loss
Kent T, Yi C, Livermore M, et al (Univ of Colorado School of Medicine, Denver)
Orthopedics 36:132-135, 2013

Lower-extremity amputations in the presence of soft tissue loss represent an unresolved conundrum because surgeons must consider sacrificing bone length to obtain adequate soft tissue coverage. Local flaps and microvascular soft tissue transfers are established strategies for maintaining residual limb length. However, the use of skin grafts remains controversial due to the presumed inferiority compared with flaps with regard to enabling prosthetic fitting and full weight bearing. The current study was designed to test the hypothesis that split-thickness skin grafts represent a safe and feasible option to preserve bone length in lower-extremity amputations with critical soft tissue loss.

▶ This article would seem to be heresy for a plastic surgeon, but the authors present enough information to suggest that, in appropriate candidates, skin grafts can provide durable end-bearing coverage for lower extremity amputations. The caveats are that the skin graft must be durable, placed on a bed of good granulation, aided by the use of ancillary vacuum-assisted tissue closure, and sensate. Finally, the prosthetic maker needs to be conversant and capable of using new materials and techniques that allow for prosthesis fitting over less-than-ideal skin. The concept is intriguing, but the study is very small (only 9 patients) and was retrospective in nature. It would be helpful to perform a prospective study and look at costs, length of time to provide usable prosthesis, and outcomes when compared with local flaps, microvascular tissue transfers, and skin grafts combined with vacuum-assisted closure.

S. H. Miller, MD

Vacuum closure as a skin-graft dressing: a comparison against conventional dressing

Petkar K, Dhanraj P, Sreekar H (CMC Vellore, Tamil Nadu)
Eur J Plast Surg 35:579-584, 2012

Background.—Grafting condition is one of the important determinants of skin-graft take. The technique of Vacuum-Closure has been claimed to improve the same and thereby graft take. However, there are few comparative studies against the conventional dressing technique evaluating its effectiveness in skin grafting. The present study was undertaken to compare Vacuum-closure with conventional dressing over freshly laid split-skin grafts.

Methods.—Consecutive patients undergoing split-skin grafting were randomized into cases and controls. The grafts in controls were covered by a conventional dressing consisting of vaseline gauze and cotton pads. Those in cases were covered by a vacuum-closure assembly and connected to a wall-suction of 80 mm Hg continuously for four days. The percentage of graft take was assessed at nine days and at two weeks and duration of the dressing were compared between the two groups. The difference in cost of the dressing was noted down.

Results.—Sixty four patients underwent split skin grafting of 71 wounds. Forty three of them were males and twenty nine were females. The grafted wounds included fresh surgically created wounds, traumatic wounds, acute and chronic burn wounds, post-inflammatory wounds and diabetic wounds. Thirty five of the grafts were cases and 36 were controls. Final graft take at two weeks in the study group ranged from 70-100 per cent with an average of 95.29 per cent graft take (SD: 5.9) while the control group showed a graft take ranging between 0-100 percent with an average graft take of 85.89 percent (SD: 25.1). Duration of dressing of the grafts was 11.63 days in cases as against 15.11 days in controls. The differences were statistically significant. The additional cost of the vacuum-closure assembly for an average sized ulcer was 6.27 pounds.

Conclusion.—Negative pressure dressing increases the amount of graft take and should be used particularly when the wound bed and grafting conditions seem less-than-ideal for a complete graft take. Negative-pressure dressing can be economically and effectively assembled using locally available materials.

Level of Evidence.—Level I, therapeutic study.

► The authors have convincingly demonstrated, as have others,[1] that negative-pressure dressings—vacuum-assisted closures (VAC)—significantly improve healing of split skin grafts. They conclude that this is particularly true when the wound bed is less than ideal, but unfortunately the size of the treated and untreated groups in their study, when broken down further into smaller groups, is such that the conclusion, although perhaps valid, reached by the data presented in this study is, in my view, insufficient. In addition, the randomization occurred after the skin graft was placed, rather than before any treatment. Was the quality of the wounds in the 2 groups really comparable so as to demonstrate that this is useful in the "difficult wound"? Were the assessments of graft take made by the surgeons performing the study and knowing which group had been treated with VAC and which not? Could the results have been strengthened by allowing an uninvolved but qualified party to make the postoperative judgments after all dressings had been removed and thus blinded to the type of treatment? Finally, the issue of increased costs was partially addressed, but a true cost/benefit analysis would have considered the increased costs for secondary treatment in the failed grafts versus that of the treated group.

S. H. Miller, MD

Reference

1. Rozen WM, Shahbaz S, Morsi A. An improved alternative to vacuum-assisted closure (VAC) as a negative pressure dressing in lower limb split skin grafting: a clinical trial. *J Plast Reconstr Aesthet Surg*. 2008;61:334-337.

Trunk and Perineal Reconstruction

A Novel Advancement Flap for Reconstruction of Massive Forehead and Temple Soft-Tissue Defects

Huang AT, Tarasidis G, Yelverton JC, et al (Virginia Commonwealth Univ, Richmond)

Laryngoscope 122:1679-1684, 2012

Objectives/Hypothesis.—To describe the authors' experience with an extended deep-plane cervicofacial (EDPCF) advancement flap, a modification of the deep-plane cervicofacial flap, for reconstruction of large forehead and temple soft-tissue defects.

Study Design.—Case series at a tertiary referral medical center.

Methods.—The charts of 11 consecutive patients who underwent EDPCF flap surgery for reconstruction of forehead and temple skin cancer defects were reviewed for demographics, smoking status, defect size, length of surgery and hospitalization, American Society of Anesthesiologists Physical Status Classification (ASA) grade, and postoperative complications.

Results.—All patients had reconstruction of large forehead and temple defects following either primary resection or Mohs micrographic surgery for skin cancer. No skin grafting was required for secondary defects. The average defect size was 52.2 cm^2. Patient ages averaged 74 years with a median ASA grade of 3. Thirty-six percent of patients admitted to smoking. Average operative time was 100 minutes, with 82% of patients treated on an outpatient basis. There were no complications of ectropion or facial nerve injury encountered. Partial distal flap necrosis occurred in one patient who admitted to smoking and resolved with conservative management.

Conclusions.—The EDCPF flap is a robust flap with a dual arterial supply and both rotation and advancement components. It is ideal in frail patients with good soft-tissue laxity and provides an immediate

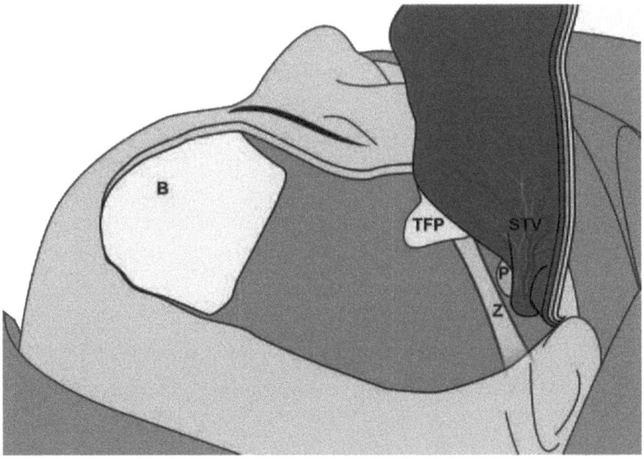

FIGURE 3.—Illustration depicting the extended deep-plane cervicofacial flap. B = bone; TFP = temporal fat pad; STV = superficial temporal vessels; P = parotid; Z = zygoma. [Color figure can be viewed in the online issue, which is available at wileyonlinelibrary.com.] (Reprinted from Huang AT, Tarasidis G, Yelverton JC, et al. A novel advancement flap for reconstruction of massive forehead and temple soft-tissue defects. *Laryngoscope*. 2012;122:1679-1684, with permission from Laryngoscope and John Wiley and Sons, www.interscience.wiley.com.)

one-stage reconstruction with ideal skin color, texture, and thickness matches for large forehead and temple defects (Fig 3).

▶ Conceptually, this type of flap was originally reported by Barton and Zilmer at the annual meeting of The American Society of Plastic Surgeons in Hawaii in 1982[1] and periodically reported in the plastic surgery literature, but primarily to repair defects of the cheek. The present authors assert that their modification—deep-plane cervicofacial dissection—makes this a safer flap for reconstruction of forehead defects, especially in smokers. However, in this small report, 1/11 patients had significant necrosis at the tip and 2 more had minor wound separation, the latter not being defined or detailed. Several other authors, including Austen et al,[2] reported virtually no difference in distal necrosis, between superficial and deep plane dissections, primarily in flaps used for check reconstruction. I believe that this flap is useful and should be considered with large cheek and forehead defects. It is an excellent flap primarily for older men, but it could also be useful in older women. I do think that when considering use of this flap in smokers or when closure of the defect is likely to be performed under a great deal of tension, one might consider flap delay to increase its hardiness and reduce the risks of distal necrosis and separation.

S. H. Miller, MD

References

1. Barton FE, Zilmer ME. The cervicofacial flap in cheek reconstruction; Anatomic and Clinical Observations presented at the annual scientific meeting of the American Society of Plastic Surgeons. 1982.

2. Austen WG, Parrett BM, Taghinia A, Wolfort SF, Upton J. The subcutaneous cervicofacial flap revisited. *Ann Plast Surg*. 2009;62:149-153.

Extremities and Trunk

The posterior tibial island flap for coverage in complex injuries of the lower extremity

Hafeez K, Siddiqui A, Rashid H-U, et al (Aga Khan Univ, Karachi, Pakistan)

Microsurgery 32:539-545, 2012

The lower third of the leg poses a surgical challenge in patients with complex injuries requiring reconstruction of soft tissue defects. The posterior tibial island fasciocutaneous flap is recognized as a suitable option for coverage of these defects, and provides a versatile solution for a complex problem. A retrospective audit was conducted at our institution from 1996 to 2008 including all patients who underwent this procedure. Patient's demographics, clinical features, outcome, and complications were noted. The study population was 24 patients (23 males, one female) with age ranging from 11 to 60 years. Mechanism of injury was road traffic accident in 20 patients and firearm injury in 4. The defect was located in the lower half of the leg in all cases. Tibial fracture was present in 15 patients, treated by external fixation in 13 and internal fixation in two patients. Fasciocutaneous flap from the medial aspect of leg was raised

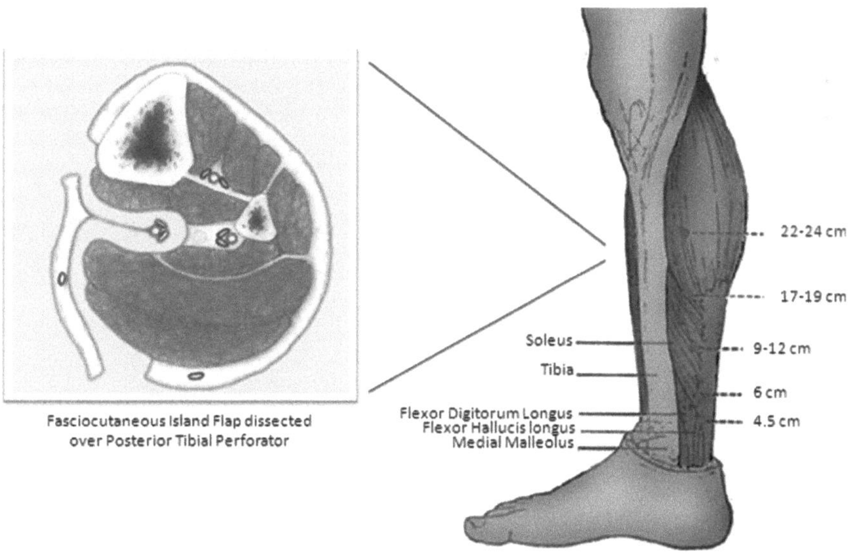

FIGURE 1.—Location of posterior tibial perforators in the leg. [Color figure can be viewed in the online issue, which is available at wileyonlinelibrary.com.] (Reprinted from Hafeez K, Siddiqui A, Rashid H-U, et al. The posterior tibial island flap for coverage in complex injuries of the lower extremity. *Microsurgery*. 2012;32:539-545, with permission from Microsurgery and Wiley-Liss, www.interscience.wiley.com.)

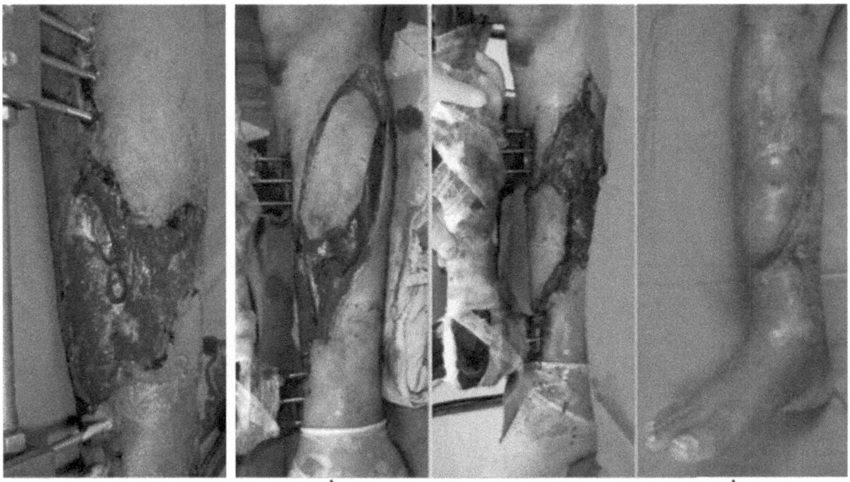

FIGURE 5.—Forty-year-old male with grade IIIB tibia fracture. (a) Defect, (b) elevation and rotation of flap, (c) split thickness skin grafting, (d) 10 months follow-up. [Color figure can be viewed in the online issue, which is available at wileyonlinelibrary.com.] (Reprinted from Hafeez K, Siddiqui A, Rashid H-U, et al. The posterior tibial island flap for coverage in complex injuries of the lower extremity. *Microsurgery.* 2012;32:539-545, with permission from Microsurgery and Wiley-Liss, www.interscience.wiley.com.)

based on a perforator of the posterior tibial artery and rotated distally. Average length of the flaps was 12.3 cm. Patients were followed for an average of 11 months (minimum 3 months). Clinical outcome was graded as good in 19 patients, fair in four patients, and poor in one patient. Posterior tibial island flap appears to be a safe and reliable option for coverage of complex wounds in lower third of the leg (Figs 1 and 5).

► This article is a worthwhile reiteration of the potential value of the posterior tibial artery fasciocutaneous flap to reconstruct moderate-to-large defects of the distal third of the leg. Of course, the key is the presence of an uninjured posterior tibial artery, an ability to include it, and the skill to include the necessary perforators in the flap. Avoiding sacrifice of the posterior tibial artery and providing a lower cost and less complex alternative to the use of free flaps for these defects are definitely pluses. In those who choose to use this type of flap, it would be most instructive to join with other centers to try to define the variables that result in complete failure or increased morbidity.

S. H. Miller, MD

Microsurgery

The Effectiveness of Pedicled Groin Flaps in the Treatment of Hand Defects: Results of 49 Patients

Goertz O, Kapalschinski N, Daigeler A, et al (Ruhr-Univ Bochum, Germany)
J Hand Surg 37A:2088-2094, 2012

Purpose.—Despite the growing number of free and local flaps used for repairing defects of the hand, groin flaps are also still widely used. The aims of this study were to evaluate the outcome of a large series of patients whose defects were covered by pedicled groin flaps, and to find out whether it is still indicated in replacing damaged soft tissue of the hand in the era of microsurgery.

Methods.—From 1982 to 2009, we treated 85 patients with soft tissue defects on the hand and distal forearm with pedicled groin flaps in our department and recorded them in a prospective database. We interviewed and examined 49 patients in this cohort.

Results.—The mean age of the 85 patients was 33 years, the male/female ratio was 4:1, the mean hospital stay was 29 ± 13 days, and the mean follow-up was 9 years. The duration to flap division was 24 ± 5 days. Altogether, we performed a mean of 4.6 operations per patient, including thinning of the flap, deepening of the interdigital fold, and stump and flap revisions. One flap loss occurred. Of the 49 patients, results were mostly classified as good, and 82% of patients would undergo the procedure again. The mean Disabilities of the Arm, Shoulder, and Hand score value was 23 ± 17. The Vancouver Scar Scale showed nearly normal height and vascularity of the groin flap (0.2 ± 0.4 and 0.3 ± 0.6, respectively), pigmentation was slightly abnormal (0.8 ± 0.6), and pliability was evaluated between "supple" and "yielding" (1.5 ± 1.2).

Conclusions.—Results achieved with the groin flaps were positive. Most patients were satisfied with the results, and the operation was easily performed when McGregor's recommendations were followed. Nevertheless, considering the high number of secondary operations, the long hospital stay, and immobilization of the arm, groin flaps should be used only when free flaps or regional pedicle flaps are either not feasible or not indicated.

Type of Study/Level of Evidence.—Therapeutic III.

► The authors present their experience with pedicled groin flaps. Their main indicators for the groin flap instead of free flap were in cases in which the patient's health is critical (eg, polytrauma), the vessels of the arm are damaged and a loop is not feasible because of a lack of soft-tissue coverage, other microsurgical interventions are likely (eg, second toe transfer), or general anesthesia and long operative time are contraindicated (eg, pregnancy). One nice operative trick is that they recommend thinning should be performed primarily, which also reduces the required distance of vessel ingrowth. This unit has an excellent microsurgery background and success rate. This makes their observations all the more interesting.

D. J. Smith, Jr, MD

Couplers in Arterial and Venous Repairs

Watson JT (Vanderbilt Univ Med Ctr, Nashville, TN)
J Hand Surg 38A:1423-1426, 2013

Background.—Atraumatic coupling of vessels of various sizes is essential to successful microvascular surgery. Traditional sutured microvascular anastomosis requires not only a steep learning curve but also time-consuming procedures, yet still can be thwarted by thrombosis and anastomosis failure. Sources of failure include intraluminal exposure of foreign material, inadequate vessel wall eversion with exposed intraluminal adventitia, uneven suture placement or cross-stitching of the lumen, luminal stenosis from imprecise bites, and tension. The development of the microvascular ring coupling device and its modifications offer the advantages of speed, intima-to-intima contact with no foreign material or adventitia interposed, and limited spasm of collapse because of the ring's stenting effect. It is also easier to handle small to moderate venous size discrepancies because "pleating" of the larger vessel into the smaller one is minimized. Patency rates range from 97% to 100%. The considerations accompanying the use of microvascular couplers in arterial and venous repairs were discussed.

Wall Structure.—Mechanical coupling in arterial repairs can be complicated by thicker wall structure, which is subject to excessive trauma and luminal stenosis after wall eversion over the metal pins. To eliminate these problems one should avoid donor and recipient luminal diameter ratios greater than 1.5:1, nonpliable vessels produced from radiation or atherosclerotic calcification, luminal diameter less than 1.5 mm, and walls too thick to be everted without injuring the intima or significantly reducing luminal diameter. More consistent success in both venous and arterial mechanical coupling is achieved with vessel diameters between 1.5 and 2.0 mm. Other complications include the erosion of suture anastomosis proficiency with greater reliance on coupling devices. Cost can also be a concern, although some researchers suggest there is a favorable cost-to-benefit ratio for mechanical coupling compared to suturing related to shorter operating room time, especially when multiple anastomoses are required.

Technical Concerns.—It is important to distribute the everted vessel wall diameter evenly among the six pins. One technique is to impale the wall on three opposite pins in a triangular configuration before positioning it on the other three pins. Selecting a ring one size less than the smaller vessel diameter in tight-fitting situations can lessen vessel wall damage. Pinching the coupler rings together after the instrument knob is removed minimizes dislodgment. Vessels should be trimmed back to healthy tissue with brisk inflow before repeat anastomosis is done. The use of more aggressive dilation of arteries to accommodate minimum ring sizes of 2.5 mm does not appear to affect patency rates in arterial walls that are less pliable. The use of 2.5-mm rings for arterial coupling may be considered a minimum if there is luminal narrowing with wall eversion over smaller rings. Small arterial lumens are common distal to the wrist and ankle. Arterial rings may not be appropriate for hand surgery, and coupling devices may cause more problems in superficial locations.

Conclusions.—Microvascular surgeons can reap benefits from using mechanical couplers in arterial and venous repairs. Significantly decreased ischemic time is one advantage. The patency rates with mechanical couplers are comparable to those found with sutured anastomoses.

▶ The author gives a brief, but relatively comprehensive, review of arterial and venous couplers. For those of you who routinely use couplers, this is not necessary reading; for those of you wanting to keep current but not using couplers, this is required reading.

D. J. Smith, Jr, MD

Factors Associated With Failed Hardware Salvage in High-Risk Patients After Microsurgical Lower Extremity Reconstruction

Patel KM, Seruya M, Franklin B, et al (Georgetown Univ Hosp, Washington, DC)

Ann Plast Surg 69:399-402, 2012

Background.—Lower extremity hardware salvage remains challenging in patients with complex comorbidities. The purpose of this study was to identify factors associated with failed hardware salvage after microsurgical lower extremity reconstruction.

Methods.—A retrospective, institutional review board-approved review was performed of patients who underwent lower extremity hardware salvage via free tissue transfer from 2004 to 2010. Outcomes were binarized into successful versus failed hardware salvage, with failure defined as nonelective removal. Patient demographics, wound characteristics, microbiology, and pathology were compared.

Results.—Thirty-four patients underwent lower extremity hardware salvage via free tissue transfer, with an average follow-up of 3.2 years (range, 0.3–7.0 years). Of these patients, 15 (44.1%) had successful hardware salvage and 19 (55.9%) required hardware removal. By demographics, a higher prevalence of multiple comorbidities was found in patients with failed hardware salvage. Wound characteristics revealed a significantly longer time to hardware coverage and longer duration of intravenous antibiotics in failed versus successful hardware salvage patients (38.9 vs 9.3 weeks, $P = 0.02$; 6.5 vs 4.1 weeks, $P = 0.03$, respectively). Initial wound cultures demonstrated a significantly higher frequency of positive growth in patients with failed versus successful hardware salvage (100.0% vs 57.1%, $P = 0.003$). Initial pathology revealed a borderline—significantly higher frequency of chronic osteomyelitis in failed versus successful salvage patients (66.7% vs 33.3%, $P = 0.08$).

Conclusions.—In this retrospective review of microsurgical lower extremity reconstruction, factors associated with failed hardware salvage included multiple comorbidities, longer time to hardware coverage, increased duration of intravenous antibiotics, positive initial wound cultures, and chronic osteomyelitis on initial pathology.

▶ The authors attempt to identify factors associated with failed hardware salvage after microsurgical lower extremity reconstruction. Although this is a retrospective study with low power, several points are worth emphasizing. Factors associated with hardware salvage included multiple comorbidities, longer time to hardware coverage, increased duration of intravenous antibiotics, positive initial wound cultures, and chronic osteomyelitis on initial pathology. Although we cannot avoid operating on these patients, keeping these factors in mind may improve the success rate, which is less than 50%. Ultimately, as the degree of wound chronicity worsens, the likelihood of successful hardware salvage decreases.

D. J. Smith, Jr, MD

Microsurgical Head and Neck Reconstruction After Oncologic Ablation: A Study Analyzing Health-Related Quality of Life

Momeni A, Kim RY, Kattan A, et al (Stanford Univ Med Ctr, Palo Alto, CA)

Ann Plast Surg 70:462-469, 2013

Background.—Evaluation of quality of life (QOL) measures is increasingly being valued as an essential parameter to determine treatment results after head and neck reconstruction. The present study was designed to evaluate the effect of microsurgical reconstruction on patient-reported QOL.

Methods.—Patients undergoing microsurgical reconstruction after radical oncosurgical ablation of head and neck malignancies from March 2007 to March 2010 were included in the study. To assess health-related QOL, the following questionnaires were sent to patients who met inclusion criteria: European Organization for Research and Treatment of Cancer (EORTC) Core Quality of Life Questionnaire (QLQ-C30 [Version 3.0]) and Head and Neck Cancer Quality of Life Questionnaire (QLQ-H and N35).

Results.—A total of 60 patients underwent microsurgical reconstruction of postablative head and neck defects during the study period. Twenty-one patients were successfully contacted, all of which completed the surveys. Satisfactory global QOL scores were achieved. Advanced age correlated with greater impairment for the ability to taste and smell ($P = 0.05$). Radiotherapy seemed to be associated with "sticky saliva"; although this was not statistically significant ($P = 0.06$). Recurrent disease at the time of surgical ablation and microsurgical reconstruction did not seem to have any appreciable impact on QOL. Finally, patients who developed postoperative complications had lower levels of "cognitive functioning" ($P = 0.04$), problems with "insomnia" ($P = 0.04$) and "social contact" ($P = 0.03$), and more commonly "felt ill" ($P = 0.03$).

Conclusions.—Improved global QOL scores were observed after microsurgical reconstruction of various head and neck defects when compared to reported pretreatment scores. Of the parameters analyzed, it seems that postoperative complications have the most profound effect on items assessed with the EORTC QLQ-C30 and H and N35 surveys. Our findings provide further scientific evidence that patients with head and neck malignancy benefit from surgical intervention with respect to postoperative QOL.

▶ The authors found improved global quality-of-life (QOL) scores after microsurgical reconstruction of various head and neck defects when compared with reported pretreatment scores. Of the parameters analyzed, postoperative complications have the most profound effect on QOL parameters. The use of QOL measures is increasingly being valued as an external parameter to determine treatment results after head and neck reconstruction. The application of QOL measures supports surgical intervention in this group of patients. Understanding the negative impact of such parameters as complications is equally important.

D. J. Smith, Jr, MD

The Evolution of Critical Concepts in Aesthetic Craniofacial Microsurgical Reconstruction

Fisher M, Dorafshar A, Bojovic B, et al (Univ of Maryland School of Medicine, Baltimore; Johns Hopkins School of Medicine, Baltimore, MD)
Plast Reconstr Surg 130:389-398, 2012

Background.—Over the last several decades, there have been numerous advances in the fields of aesthetic, craniofacial, and microsurgery. Aesthetic units are no longer "skin deep" but are recognized as being composed of both soft and hard tissue. Indeed, hard tissue must complement the soft tissue to recreate the unit. In addition, revisionary procedures have become necessary to achieve the desired result. Here, the authors integrate seven critical concepts and provide a patient series illustrating their success.

Methods.—The authors assembled a two-center, retrospective cohort review of patients who underwent free-tissue transfer of craniofacial defects at the R Adams Cowley Shock Trauma Center and the Johns Hopkins Hospital from 2003 to 2011. Patients were categorized by anatomic location, complications recorded, and illustrative cases selected.

Results.—A total of 184 patients with craniofacial defects were identified: 79 female and 105 male patients, with a mean age of 44 years. Etiologies included cancer (51.6 percent), trauma (39.1 percent), congenital defects (6.5 percent), and infection (2.7 percent). Free-tissue transfers included 67 fibula, 42 anterolateral thigh, 41 ulnar, 18 groin, 14 iliac, three radius, and one vastus lateralis flaps. The success rate was 97.3 percent and complication rate was 10.8 percent. Secondary procedures included suction lipectomy, dermabrasion, tissue resuspension, and cutaneous flap excision followed by full-thickness skin grafting or tissue rearrangement.

Conclusions.—To achieve aesthetically pleasing results in free-flap facial reconstruction, the authors define seven critical concepts to guide the reconstruction: aesthetic-unit appearance, defect boundaries, tissue requirements, vascularized skeletal buttress framework, ample soft-tissue volume, early reconstruction, and local revisional procedures.

Clinical Question/Level of Evidence.—Therapeutic, IV.

▶ The authors present the evolution of the refinements of their techniques in craniofacial reconstruction. Key to this understanding is the recognition that aesthetic units are no longer "skin deep" and are recognized as being composed of both soft and hard tissue. Advances in aesthetic, craniofacial, and microsurgery have all contributed. Ultimately, the authors define seven critical concepts to guide the reconstruction: aesthetic-unit appearance, defect boundaries, tissue requirements, vascularized skeletal buttress framework, ample soft-tissue volume, early reconstruction, and local revisional procedures. Manson and Rodriguez have a wealth of experience in this area, and this article is a must for anyone working in this clinical area.

D. J. Smith, Jr, MD

Achieving Aesthetic Results in Facial Reconstructive Microsurgery: Planning and Executing Secondary Refinements

Haddock NT, Saadeh PB, Siebert JW (New York Univ Langone Med Ctr; Univ of Wisconsin, Madison)

Plast Reconstr Surg 130:1236-1245, 2012

Background.—Free tissue transfer to improve bulk and contour in facial deformities has been proven useful, yet refinements that turn an acceptable result into an excellent result are essential to reconstruction. The authors reviewed their experience and described these refinements.

Methods.—The charts of 371 free tissue transfer cases (1989 to 2010) performed by the senior author (J.W.S.) were reviewed. Free tissue transfer of a circumflex scapular variant flap or superficial inferior epigastric was performed to treat deformities arising from hemifacial atrophy ($n = 126$), hemifacial microsomia ($n = 89$), radiation therapy ($n = 40$), bilateral malformations including lupus and polymyositis ($n = 50$), other congenital anomalies ($n = 25$), facial palsy ($n = 17$), and burns and trauma ($n = 24$).

Results.—Revision surgery planning began at initial flap operation where the flap was stretched maximally and interdigitated with recipient tissue. More tissue was required in the malar region. Revision refinement was indicated in all cases (after 6 months). Flap revision involved liposuction, debulking, reelevation, and release of tethering, followed by tissue rearrangement by means of advancement, rotation, transposition, and/or turnover flaps of subcutaneous tissues from the previous free flap. The jawline frequently required more debulking. Periorbital reconstruction was combined with lower lid support with or without canthal repositioning. Conventional face-lift techniques with the flap as superficial musculoaponeurotic system augmented the result. Autologous fat injection to the alar rim, medial canthus, upper eyelid, and lip was a useful adjunct. Severe lip deficiencies were addressed with local flaps.

Conclusion.—The keys to improving results were continual critical reassessment, open-mindedness to new approaches, and maintaining high expectations.

Clinical Question/Level of Evidence.—Therapeutic, V.

▶ The senior author has a long history with free tissue transfer to improve bulk and contour in facial deformities. In this article, the authors describe their experience and their refinements to turn an acceptable result into an excellent result. Particularly helpful is Fig 1 in the original article, which outlines lessons learned and standardization of surgical approach. Further, patient satisfaction significantly improved with revision surgery. Revision surgery is basically begun as part of the initial planning. This is a must-read article for all, even those not doing microsurgery. It addresses a difficult problem and shows how, with careful analysis and planning, improvement can be made.

D. J. Smith, Jr, MD

Microsurgical Repair of the Inferior Alveolar Nerve: Success Rate and Factors That Adversely Affect Outcome

Bagheri SC, Meyer RA, Cho SH, et al (Northside Hosp, Atlanta, GA; Georgia Oral and Facial Surgery, Marietta; Emory Univ School of Medicine, Atlanta, GA)
J Oral Maxillofac Surg 70:1978-1990, 2012

Purpose.—The objectives of this study were to determine the likelihood of regaining functional sensory recovery (FSR) after microsurgical repair of the inferior alveolar nerve (IAN), and which variables significantly affected the outcome of that surgery in a large series of patients.

Materials and Methods.—This was a retrospective cohort study that evaluated all patients who had undergone microsurgical repair of the IAN by 1 of the senior surgeons (R.A.M.) from March 1986 through December 2005. The requirements for inclusion of a patient in the study included the availability of a complete chart record and a final follow-up visit at least 12 months after surgery. All other patients were excluded. The predictor variables were categorized as demographic, etiologic, and operative. The final outcome variable was the level of recovery of sensory function as determined by standardized neurosensory testing at the last postoperative visit of each patient and based on guidelines established by the Medical Research Council Scale. Risk factors for surgical failure to achieve useful sensory function were determined from analysis of descriptive statistics, including patient age, patient gender, etiology of nerve injury, chief sensory complaint (numbness, pain, or both), time from injury to surgical intervention (in months), intraoperative findings, and surgical procedure. Logistic regression methods and associated odds ratios were used to quantify the association between the risk factors and improvement. Receiver operator characteristic curve analysis was used to find the threshold of those variables that significantly affected patient outcome.

Results.—In total, 167 patients (41 male and 126 female patients; mean age, 38.7 years [range, 15-75 years]) underwent 186 IAN repairs (19 patients sustained bilateral IAN injuries). The mean time from injury until surgery was 10.7 months (range, 0-72 months). Successful recovery from neurosensory dysfunction (FSR, defined by the Medical Research Council Scale as ranging from useful sensory function to complete sensory recovery) was observed in 152 repaired IANs (81.7%). With increasing duration from date of injury to IAN repair, the likelihood of FSR decreased (odds ratio, 0.898; $P < .001$). The odds of achieving FSR exhibited a linear decline between the date of nerve injury and its repair, with a significant drop in rate of successful outcome (FSR) occurring beginning at 12 months after injury. There was also a significant negative relationship between increasing patient age and improvement (odds ratio, 0.97; $P = .015$), with a threshold drop of achieving FSR at 51 years of age. The cause of the injury, the operative findings, and the type of operation performed to repair the nerve had no significant effect on the likelihood of the patient regaining FSR. The presence of pain after nerve injury did not affect the likelihood of achieving FSR after repair in a statistically significant manner ($P = .08$). In those patients who did not have pain as a major complaint before nerve repair, pain did not develop after microneurosurgery.

Conclusions.—Microsurgical repair of an IAN injury resulted in successful restoration of an acceptable level of neurosensory function (FSR) in most patients (152 of 186 repairs [81.7%]) in this study. The likelihood of regaining FSR was inversely related to both time between the injury and its repair and increasing patient age, with significant threshold drops at 12 months after nerve injury and at 51 years of age, respectively.

▶ Over the past 6 months, I have received 2 referrals for inferior alveolar nerve injury. I admit to not being as well versed as I should about this subject, so this article is included. The authors report successful recovery from neurosensory dysfunction (functional sensory recovery [FSR]) in 81.7% of repaired inferior alveolar nerves. The chance of successful FSR decreases with increasing time from injury, especially after 12 months. All other factors affecting successful nerve repairs seem to apply to the inferior alveolar nerve. It makes sense that we should more aggressively look for and manage these patients.

D. J. Smith, Jr, MD

A Review of Microvascular Ear Replantation

Jung SW, Lee J, Oh SJ, et al (Hallym Univ Med Ctr, Anyang-si, Republic of Korea; et al)

J Reconstr Microsurg 29:181-188, 2013

Microvascular ear replantation is a significant challenge because of the small size of the vessels and the fact that traumatic amputations are frequently avulsed. The zone of trauma is therefore extended and the primary repair of the injured vessel is rendered unlikely. The purpose of this study is to review the literature of ear replantation. A review of the relevant literature that has been published since 1980 revealed 47 cases reported in 37 publications. We present 5 cases from our own experience and analyze a total 52 cases of microvascular ear replantation. The patient's age, sex, degree of amputation, cause of injury, ischemic time, method of arterial and venous anastomosis, complications, any additional outflow used, postoperative medications, the requirement for transfusions, and the number of hospital admission days are described. Successful microvascular ear replantations require anastomosis of the vessels if possible. Rather than a vein graft, primary repair of the vessels, or at least pedicled repair of the artery, should be considered to ensure flap survival. In addition, vein repair should be considered if possible to ensure the secure drainage of blood from the replant. With secure circulation, the replant can survive, resulting in a very satisfactory outcome.

▶ Although rare, ear replantation does occur with some regularity. These authors add 5 cases to the already reported 47. They note that review of the series is only on successful replantations, not failures, which certainly might skew the data. Interestingly, survival with no venous repair (64.7%) is comparable to survival with venous repair (62.9%). The authors' technical contribution is summarized in 3 main points: (1) minimal debridement to avoid damage to normal vascular tissue, (2) primary repair as the preferred choice, and (3) use of 11-0 nylon suture. Although not an in-depth or exhaustive review, this is very informative for anyone who does replantation surgery. Without a doubt, immediate microvascular ear replantation remains the preferred method for ear reconstruction.

D. J. Smith, Jr, MD

Microvascular approach to scalp replantation and reconstruction: A thirty-six year experience

Herrera F, Buntic R, Brooks D, et al (California Pacific Med Ctr, San Francisco)

Microsurgery 32:591-597, 2012

Background.—Soft tissue defects of the scalp may result from multiple etiologies and can be challenging to reconstruct. We discuss our experience with scalp replantation and secondary microvascular reconstruction over 36 years, including techniques pioneered at our institution with twin–twin scalp allotransplant and innervated partial superior latissimus dorsi (LD) for scalp/frontalis loss.

Methods.—A retrospective review of all patients presenting with scalp loss requiring microvascular reconstruction at a single center was performed from January 1971 to January 2007. Medical records were reviewed for age, gender, defect size/location, etiology, type of reconstruction, recipient vessels used, vein grafts, and complications.

Results.—Thirty-three patients were identified; mean age was 33 years (range, 7–79). Mean scalp defect size was 442 cm^2 (range, 120–900 cm^2). Thirty-six microvascular reconstructions were performed; of these, 10 scalp replants and 26 microvascular tissue transfers. Of these 26, 17 were LD based (partial superior LD with and without reinnervation, LD combined with serratus, LD combined with parascapular, LD combined with split rib, LD only) and 2 free scalp allotransplant among others. The superficial temporal artery and vein was used as recipient vessels in 70% of cases. Overall, microvascular success rate was 92%; complications occurred in 14 cases, nine major (tumor recurrence [$n = 2$], partial flap loss [$n = 2$], replant loss [$n = 3$, size <300 cm^2], hematoma [$n = 2$]) and five minor (donor site seroma /hematoma [$n = 3$], flap congestion [$n = 1$], superficial wound infection [$n = 1$]).

Conclusions.—Every attempt should be made at scalp replantation when the patient is stable and the parts salvageable. Larger avulsion defects had higher success rates after replantation than smaller defects (<300 cm^2), with the superficial temporal artery and vein most commonly used for recipient vessels ($P = 0.0083$). Microvascular tissue transfer remains a mainstay of treatment for scalp defects, with LD-based flaps, demonstrating excellent versatility for a range of defects.

► Any time a major center presents its experience with a particular procedure, it is worth reviewing. In this case, the Buncke Clinic reviews their 36-year experience with scalp replantation and reconstruction. This is certainly the largest experience reported in the literature. It is worth reviewing by anyone doing this type of surgery, but it is disappointing that no major nuances are identified.

D. J. Smith, Jr, MD

7 Miscellaneous

General

Applicability of Large Databases in Outcomes Research

Malay S, Shauver MJ, Chung KC (The Univ of Michigan Med School, Ann Arbor)

J Hand Surg 37A:1437-1446, 2012

Outcomes research serves as a mechanism to assess the quality of care, cost effectiveness of treatment, and other aspects of health care. The use of administrative databases in outcomes research is increasing in all medical specialties, including hand surgery. However, the real value of databases can be maximized with a thorough understanding of their contents, advantages, and limitations. We performed a literature review pertaining to databases in medical, surgical, and epidemiologic research, with special emphasis on orthopedic and hand surgery. This article provides an overview of the available database resources for outcomes research, their potential value to hand surgeons, and suggestions to improve their effective use.

▶ Outcomes research serves as a mechanism to assess the quality of care, cost-effectiveness of treatment, and other aspects of health care. Using administrative databases in outcomes research is increasing in all medical specialties. The real value of databases can only be maximized with a thorough understanding of their contents, advantages, and limitations. The authors performed a literature review pertaining to databases in medical, surgical, and epidemiologic research, with special emphasis on orthopedic and hand surgery. This article provides an overview of the available database resources for outcomes research, their potential value to hand surgeons, and suggestions to improve their effective use. This is an excellent overview and a must-read for anyone wanting to stay current in outcomes research.

D. J. Smith, Jr, MD

Latent Class Analysis

Neuhaus V, Ring DC (Massachusetts General Hosp, Boston)
J Hand Surg 38A:1018-1020, 2013

Background.—Gold standard or reference tests do not exist for all diseases or disorders. In the absence of a reference standard, latent class analysis (LCA) is being used increasingly. In LDA, unobserved (or latent) associations of risk factors that estimate the probability of disease are identified.

Methods and Limitations.—The relationship between variable A and variable B may be spurious and mediated by an undetected variable (X). Using data collected for variables A and B, LCA estimates the profile of X and calculates the number of meaningful classes for X using probability calculations. A variety of best model fits can be used to identify the ideal number of classes. These best model fits identify the goodness of fit as well as the information lost with the various models when a number of classes has been determined. With the ideal number of classes known, LCA allows one to calculate the probability for the presence of disease in each class. Accuracy is determined by comparing the results of a new test method for X with the probabilities calculated for these classes of variables.

The unrestricted LCA model requires three or more independent and clinically meaningful categorical variables with at least binary data. If the sample size is small, variables are correlated or continuous, and probability is small or large, the probability estimate in distinct latent classes can yield overestimates or underestimates. LCA also requires special software.

Applications.—LCA has been applied in two main ways: (1) to identify meaningful subgroups of patients who may benefit from targeted treatment, especially with respect to pain, and (2) to validate new classification systems, diagnostic criteria, or tests. LCA-based tests or systems show better agreement and accuracy in detecting outcomes or disease.

Conclusions.—LCA offers the means for statistically analyzing meaningful but often subtle groups of patient factors that may correlate with disease probabilities. It can estimate the accuracy of diagnosis when no reference standard exists. It allows a more scientific approach to areas that are often nebulous for practitioners. LCA helps patients and clinicians become more comfortable with the inherent and possibly unavoidable limitations of diagnosis and treatment.

▶ The gold or reference standard is a valid or reliable test that can make a diagnosis with certainty. In the absence of a reference standard, an increasingly used statistical method is latent class analysis (LCA), which identifies unobserved (or latent) associations of risk factors that estimate the probability of disease. LCA allows us to be scientific about some of the nebulous aspects referred to as "the art of medicine." If you are not familiar with LCA, this is an excellent preview; if you are, this is an excellent quick review.

D. J. Smith, Jr, MD

The Level of Evidence Presented at Plastic Surgery Meetings: What Do We Have to Learn?

Chuback JE, Varley TL, Yarascavitch BA, et al (McMaster Univ, Hamilton, Ontario, Canada; Univ of North Carolina, Charlotte)

Plast Reconstr Surg 131:776-783, 2013

Background.—Internationally, plastic surgery societies have placed an increasing emphasis on the importance of evidence-based medicine. The authors aimed to categorize levels of evidence of podium presentations at three major North American plastic surgical meetings, and to assess the factors associated with a higher level evidence.

Methods.—Presentations at the 2010/2011 meetings of three of the largest societies of plastic surgeons in North America were evaluated for the area of research, number and origin of authors, subdomain of plastic surgery, number of centers of collaboration, number of subjects, study subtype, and level of evidence.

Results.—One hundred eighty-eight presentations were screened, and 126 met eligibility criteria. The American Society of Plastic Surgeons was the largest meeting with 74 presentations (58.7 percent). Breast (23.8 percent) and craniofacial (21.4 percent) topics were most frequently covered. Most studies had five or fewer authors (76.4 percent), were conducted at a single center (84.3 percent), were therapeutic (89.7 percent), and had 50 or fewer subjects (36.8 percent). Two studies (1.6 percent) were level I, 11 (8.7 percent) were level II, 54 (42.9 percent) were level III, 46 (36.5 percent) were level IV, and 13 (10.3 percent) were level V. Overall, the mean level of evidence was 3.45, and one of every 10 presentations was of higher level of evidence (level I or II). Higher level evidence presentations were found to be associated with multicenter studies.

Conclusions.—Evidence presented at major plastic surgical meetings is rarely level I and infrequently level II. Opportunities to create greater awareness of the need for prospective high-level studies are needed.

► Educational meetings frequently highlight the latest innovations and cutting-edge treatments, with much of the content not yet peer reviewed. As this article reminds us, most of what is presented is not based on high- or low-quality prospective or comparative studies, or on systematic reviews, but rather on lesser-quality retrospective cohort or comparative studies or large case series. Proper interpretation of conclusions and actual implementation into practice should be tempered by the limitations of lower-level (III, IV, and IV) studies.

K. A. Gutowski, MD

The Evils of Nicotine: An Evidence-Based Guide to Smoking and Plastic Surgery

Rinker B (Univ of Kentucky College of Medicine, Lexington)
Ann Plast Surg 70:599-605, 2013

As nearly 1 of 5 adult Americans are smokers, plastic surgeons should be familiar with the effect of smoking on perioperative risk, the importance of smoking cessation, and the tools to help patients quit. Cigarette smoke contains over 250 known toxins, including nicotine, carbon monoxide, hydrogen cyanide, and nitric oxide, which all are known to impair wound healing, through multiple mechanisms. The relationship of smoking and delayed postoperative wound healing has been established in numerous prospective and retrospective cohort studies (level 2 and 3 evidence), and has been demonstrated across a wide range of surgical disciplines and procedures, including many common plastic surgical procedures. The ameliorating effects of cessation are supported by level 1 evidence, which suggests that the optimal duration of preoperative cessation is 4 weeks or longer. Nicotine replacement therapy and smoking cessation medications are effective aids for quitting and should be familiar to plastic surgeons.

▶ According to a survey, most plastic surgeons will have their patients stop smoking 2 weeks before surgery. However, based on well-done studies, the ideal time of cessation before surgery seems to be at least 4 weeks and may be 6 weeks or more. There is level 1 and 2 evidence that active smoking increases the risk of postoperative wound infection and delayed wound healing by 2- to 3-fold.

Specific plastic surgery procedures, such as facelift, abdominoplasty, and breast reconstruction with implants, should be considered high-risk procedures in active smokers, with a pooled relative risk greater than 3 for wound healing complications. Autologous breast reconstruction and breast reduction should be considered a moderate risk with a pooled relative risk between 2 and 3. In free tissue transfers to the head and neck, smokers were found to have an elevated risk for wound healing complications but not for flap loss.

Medication and physician counseling can double the chance of successful smoking cessation, and urine cotinine testing is an effective, inexpensive, and underused method to confirm cessation. When offering patients a way to stop smoking before surgery, nicotine replacement therapy (NRT) may be a good option, as a randomized, clinical trial showed that smoking cessation with NRT reduced postoperative wound healing complications as much as smoking cessation alone.

K. A. Gutowski, MD

The Use of Prophylactic Antibiotics in Plastic Surgery: Update in 2010
Hauck RM, Nogan S (Penn State Univ, Hershey, PA)
Ann Plast Surg 70:91-97, 2013

Background.—The indications for prophylactic antibiotics in plastic surgery remain controversial. No recent survey has been reported on the use of prophylactic antibiotics by plastic surgeons in clinical practice. This survey was designed to assess the current use of prophylactic antibiotics by plastic surgeons and to compare trends with previous studies.

Methods.—All members of the American Society of Plastic Surgeons with an e-mail address on the Society's website were contacted via an e-mail and sent a link to a SurveyMonkey questionnaire. To survey only in those subspecialty areas that they practice in, surgeons were queried only on the procedures that they perform. Within each section, a list of common representative procedures was included, with questions about the use of antibiotic prophylaxis.

Results.—A total of 3824 American Society of Plastic Surgeons members were contacted. Of the 3613, 910 with working e-mail addresses responded to the survey for a response rate of 25%. And 833 or 91.5% completed the survey. Survey data cover the percentage of surgeons reporting their use of antibiotics in procedures that they currently perform. The percentage of plastic surgeons who use prophylactic antibiotics in almost all procedures studied has increased significantly when compared with earlier studies.

Conclusions.—The use of prophylactic antibiotics by plastic surgeons has increased considerably since the prior studies by Krizek et al (*Plast Reconstr Surg*. 1975;55:21–32 and 1985;76:953–963). Some of these uses are appropriate because of the use in procedures involving implants and longer operations. The elevated rates for clean procedures are not part of the evidence-based practice.

▶ Recent quality improvement efforts by government agencies, professional organizations, and hospitals have tried to reduce unnecessary antibiotic use while measuring the appropriateness of prophylactic antibiotics for surgical procedures. In most aesthetic surgery cases, there is no need for prophylactic antibiotics beyond those given intravenously within an hour of incision (and repeated after 4 hours in longer cases) even if implants are used or drains are left in place. Based on the findings of this survey, many plastic surgeons need to rethink their overuse of prophylactic antibiotics.

K. A. Gutowski, MD

Are We Too Cavalier About Antiviral Prophylaxis?

Onwudiwe OC, Marmur ES, Cohen JL (AllPhases Dermatology, Alexandria, VA; Mount Sinai School of Medicine, NY; About-Skin Dermatology and DermSurgery, Englewood, CO)

J Drugs Dermatol 12:199-205, 2013

Herpes simplex virus (HSV) prophylaxis may be underutilized in cosmetic surgery at a time when cosmetic procedures are increasing. Our goal is to review the data regarding HSV prophylaxis in order to remind cosmetic surgeons when to consider adding this regimen to their patient perioperative care.

▶ Herpes simplex virus (HSV) has been reported after procedures such as laser resurfacing, dermabrasion, chemical peels, Mohs surgery, and dermal filler injections. In procedures in which the skin is either completely de-epithelialized or dramatically altered, pathognomonic signs of HSV infection may not develop, and the diagnosis of HSV can be difficult, as there is often no apparent difference between the presentation of bacterial, fungal, or viral infections on denuded skin. Irritant contact dermatitis after skin resurfacing can also present with painful erosions, mimicking HSV reactivation. Infections of these areas typically occur between 3 and 10 days after the procedure and present with fragile vesicles or pustules that can progress into erosions. Viral infections can delay healing and lead to secondary bacterial infection and, subsequently, scarring.

The following recommendations are based on the authors' review of the literature. To date, there are no standard protocols outlining who should receive prophylaxis, the duration of treatment, and the drug of choice.

1. Culture all suspected infected lesions for bacterial, viral, and fungal etiologies (de-epithelialized wounds can lead to confusing appearances and may not have their characteristic morphology and, thus, can look alike).
2. Antiviral prophylaxis should be given to any patient with a strong history of herpes outbreaks who is undergoing cutaneous procedures that involve deeper penetration into the skin—especially when the perioral area is part of the treatment region (laser resurfacing, fractionated laser procedures, dermabrasion, medium to deeper chemical peels, fillers/soft tissue augmentation, and skin cancer reconstruction).
3. Procedures with limited potential injury (superficial peels, microdermabrasion, and botulinum toxin injections) can be excluded as long as there is no sign of recent HSV infection.
4. Any person undergoing full-face or perioral laser resurfacing or medium to deep full-face chemical peels, regardless of a negative history, should receive prophylaxis.
5. All immunocompromised patients should be strongly considered to receive antiviral prophylaxis for facial procedures regardless of their known history of HSV infection.
6. Prophylaxis should be strongly considered in patients receiving dermal fillers in the perioral area, full-face or near full-face photodynamic therapy,

skin cancer excisions and Mohs surgery repairs with extensive undermining or flap formation (especially in the V2/V3 region), perioral laser resurfacing, and perioral medium to deep chemicals.

7. Prophylaxis should be continued at least until full re-epithelialization has occurred, which typically takes 7 to 10 days. Because viral infection can erupt after re-epithelialization, treatment must be continued at least a few days after that.
8. Prophylaxis may be started the day before or the morning of the procedure (no significant difference in the number of outbreaks with either regimen).
9. In terms of selecting a prophylactic antiviral agent, immunosuppression, tolerability and safety, bioavailability, and cost should be considered. Options include acyclovir, valacyclovir, and famciclovir.

K. A. Gutowski, MD

Current Trends in Chaperone Use by Plastic and Reconstructive Surgeons

Choudry U, Barta RJ, Kim N (Univ of Minnesota, Minneapolis; Med College of Wisconsin, Milwaukee)

Ann Plast Surg 70:709-713, 2013

Purpose.—There is a paucity of literature regarding the use of chaperones by surgeons when examining patients. Use of a chaperone not only makes the patient comfortable but also potentially protects the surgeon from perceived misconduct. This is especially true for plastic surgeons who examine sensitive areas commonly. The purpose of this study was to determine the current trends in chaperone use by plastic surgeons when examining patients.

Materials and Methods.—A 23-question online survey was sent to all members of the American Society of Plastic Surgeons. Data collected online were analyzed using Student t test and Pearson χ^2 test. A $P < 0.05$ was considered significant.

Results.—Of the 4990 surgeons polled, 830 (16.6%) responded to some or all of the questions (707 [85%] male; 117 [14%] female). The overall chaperone use by plastic surgeons during all examinations of patients was 30%. This rate increased up to 60% while examining sensitive areas. Male surgeons reported a higher frequency of chaperone use than female surgeons ($P < 0.001$). Cosmetic surgeons had a higher rate of chaperone use compared to reconstructive surgeons ($P = 0.001$). Similarly, surgeons who had been in practice for more than 20 years reported a higher rate of chaperone use compared to surgeons in practice for less than 20 years ($P = 0.032$). Sixty-one (7.6%; 56 male and 5 female) surgeons reported being accused of inappropriate behavior by patients, of whom 49 (80%) did not have a chaperone present. There was no significant difference among male and female surgeons in rates of being accused of inappropriate behavior (7.9% vs 4.2%, $P = 0.19$).

Conclusions.—There was a higher rate of chaperone use by male plastic surgeons, surgeons with more than 20 years experience, and cosmetic surgeons. Despite the difference in chaperone use between the sexes, both had similar rates of being accused of inappropriate behavior during examinations by patients, and although these incidents were quite low, most had no chaperone present during those examinations.

▶ Having a chaperone present during a patient encounter when sensitive areas are examined is prudent, particularly when 1 of 13 plastic surgeons reported being accused of inappropriate behavior by a patient. However, there is no standard of care, and neither professional societies nor hospitals offer guidelines for such situations. In many practices, the additional costs and the interruption of workflow make regular use of a chaperone difficult to implement.

K. A. Gutowski, MD

The Management of Postoperative Nausea and Vomiting: Current Thoughts and Protocols

Sweis I, Yegiyants SS, Cohen MN (Univ of Chicago, IL)

Aesthetic Plast Surg 37:625-633, 2013

The postoperative course of surgical patients can have a tremendous impact on the surgical outcome and on patient satisfaction. One of the most significant issues is postoperative nausea and vomiting (PONV) which, despite being a common side effect of general anesthesia, has received little attention in the plastic surgery literature. The incidence and potential consequences of PONV are frequently underestimated and consequently the need for prophylaxis is often overlooked. There are significant consequences to this seemingly minor morbidity that extend beyond patient discomfort and dissatisfaction. In addition to being considered a significant undesirable outcome by patients, severe cases of PONV may result in postoperative complications and unplanned hospital admissions. In this article we overview the mechanism, pathophysiology, and risk factors for PONV and provide a comprehensive algorithmic approach to its management.

Level of Evidence V.—This journal requires that authors assign a level of evidence to each article. For a full description of these Evidence-Based Medicine ratings, please refer to the Table of Contents or the online Instructions to Authors www.springer.com/00266.

▶ As more procedures are done in an ambulatory surgery setting, prevention and treatment of postoperative nausea and vomiting (PONV) have gained attention. For aesthetic surgery patients, PONV not only contributes to an unsatisfactory experience and delays in being discharged to home but can increase bleeding and hematoma formation, cause strain on tissue repairs, and result in skin closure dehiscence. In severe cases, hospitalization for dehydration and metabolic imbalances may result.

The Apfel score is commonly used as a risk assessment tool for PONV. Factors for increased PONV are female gender, a history of motion sickness, being a nonsmoker, and use of perioperative opioids.

The presence of 0, 1, 2, 3, or 4 of these factors correlates to a PONV incidence of 10%, 21%, 39%, 61%, and 79%, respectively. Patient prophylaxis based on these Apfel scores has been shown to lead to a decreased incidence of PONV. Other risk factors include history of PONV, young age, obesity, anxiety, surgery lasting more than 3 hours, breast surgery, facial rejuvenation surgery, and use of general anesthesia.

Effective prevention and management of PONV includes risk assessment for developing PONV and baseline risk reduction, PONV prophylaxis and use of cost-effective PONV treatment, and a combination of PONV therapy and rescue treatment. Plastic surgeons should be familiar with this review paper.

K. A. Gutowski, MD

The use of platelet-rich plasma in plastic surgery: A systematic review

Sommeling CE, Heyneman A, Hoeksema H, et al (Ghent Univ Hosp, Belgium)

J Plast Reconstr Aesthet Surg 66:301-311, 2013

Objective.—The study's aim was to evaluate the available evidence regarding the use of platelet-rich plasma in plastic and reconstructive surgery, through implementation of a systematic review of the literature.

Data Sources.—PubMed and The Cochrane Library were searched using MeSH terms: 'platelet rich plasma' and 'plastic surgery' for all publications up to July 2011. All English, German, French and Dutch papers were included. In addition, the reference lists of relevant articles were searched for potentially appropriate publications.

Study Selection.—Included studies needed to report on topics related to plastic and reconstructive surgery, mentioning at least one clinical end point. Both *in vivo* and *in vitro* comparative studies, performed in humans or animals, were included. A total of 82 publications were found, of which 40 studies met the inclusion criteria and were relevant to be used in this systematic review.

Data Extraction.—Data from retrieved studies were reviewed and tabulated according to year of publication, study design, human or animal studies, characteristics of the population, mode of application, outcomes and preparation method.

Data Synthesis.—A total of 15 randomised controlled trials and 25 case–control studies were found. Thirty-six publications demonstrated favourable outcomes with the use of platelet-rich plasma. The included articles were divided into three topics related to plastic surgery: wound healing, fat grafting and bone grafting.

Conclusions.—This systematic review describes a substantially beneficial effect of platelet-rich plasma for several indications, including a better wound healing rate, an increased survival rate of fat grafts and an enhancement of bone graft regeneration.

▶ Platelet-rich plasma (PRP) is the portion of the plasma fraction of autologous blood that has a platelet concentration above baseline values. It is formed by centrifugation of whole blood (drawn from a peripheral vein), which separates the various components of blood by their specific weight and increases the concentration of platelets. Under normal conditions (wound creation), activated platelets release cytokines and growth factors (GF) shortly after clotting. This can also be done by using an activator (thrombin), resulting in the formation of a platelet gel that acts as a drug delivery system because of its high concentration of platelets and their active cytokines and growth factors, which stimulate physiologic processes. Platelet synthesis of platelet-derived GF, transforming GF-beta-1, vascular endothelial GF, and epidermal GF are considered to be the most important in local tissue repair and regrowth.

PRP has gained popularity in orthopedic medicine to treat degenerative conditions and accelerate healing of injured tissue. The regenerative properties are being promoted in plastic surgery for both reconstructive and aesthetic purposes at a pace that exceeds well-done clinical trials supporting its use. Based on this article, 3 of 6 randomized, controlled trials found a statistically significant improvement in human wound healing attributed to PRP application. Animal studies showed new capillary formation with fibroblastic and endothelial cell proliferation.

Fat grafting with PRP was done in 5 case-controlled clinical studies. When PRP was used, 3 studies showed decreased time to wound healing and 1 showed enhancement of facial fat graft volume after 1 year. However, 1 study found no effect in breast fat grafting and another study did not show a reduction in the number of fat grafting sessions (but did see more fat necrosis). Two of 4 animal studies showed improved fat grafting when PRP was used.

Based on this systematic study, there is evidence that PRP possesses a beneficial effect for tissue healing and possibly cellular therapies. However, consistent evidence concerning the clinical applications of PRP is lacking, perhaps because of a lack of standardized protocols or patient selection. Until more well-designed clinical studies are available, it is hard to recommend PRP treatments for aesthetic applications.

K. A. Gutowski, MD

Tissue Expanders

Effects of hyperbaric oxygen therapy on rapid tissue expansion in rabbits

Ju Z, Wei J, Guan H, et al (Fourth Military Med Univ, Shannxi, PR China)
J Plast Reconstr Aesthet Surg 65:1252-1258, 2012

Background.—Tissue expansion has been widely used to provide additional soft tissue for clinical reconstruction. Rapid expansion requires a much shorter clinical period than conventional expansion; however, less natural skin growth occurs resulting in a larger stretch-back ratio and insufficient extra soft tissue for clinical use. In this study, hyperbaric oxygen therapy (HBOT) was used in the inflation phase of rapid expansion to increase natural skin growth.

Methods.—Twelve rabbits were divided into two groups. Each group received rapid expander inflation every day. One group received HBOT and the other did not. Blood flow in the expanded skin of each rabbit was assayed in the 10-day inflation phase. After the inflation phase, a rectangular expanded flap of each rabbit was harvested. The instant stretch-back ratio, tension, weight and histological characteristics of the flaps were evaluated.

Results.—(1) After the second inflation day, the mean blood flow of the HBOT group became significantly higher than that of the control with each day ($P < 0.05$). At the last day, the blood flow of the HBOT group increased to 131 ± 17 pu, while the control group decreased to 35 ± 5 pu. (2) The mean instant stretch-back ratio of the HBOT group under no-tension conditions was 29 ± 4%, which was significantly less than that of the control group, 46 ± 3% ($P < 0.01$). (3) The mean flap tension of the HBOT group was 15.3000 ± 1.47648 g and 12.9833 ± 0.73598 g in the transverse and longitudinal axis, respectively, both significantly smaller than that of the control group (33.9167 ± 4.78390 g and 26.5000 ± 2.45031 g, respectively) ($P < 0.01$). (4) Mean per unit flap weight of the HBOT group was 0.221 ± 0.005 g cm^{-2}, significantly heavier ($P < 0.01$) than that of the control group (0.143 ± 0.010 g cm^{-2}). (5) Histologically, the epidermal layer and thickness of the expanded skin of the HBOT group were much thicker than those of the control group, and more vessels were visible in the subcutaneous tissue.

Conclusions.—The use of HBOT in the inflation phase of rapid expansion can effectively promote blood flow in the expanded skin, increase its natural skin growth and reduce the instant stretch-back ratio and tension of expanded skin.

▶ This is a Fascinating fascinating early study in a rabbit model demonstrating the salubrious effects of hyperbaric oxygen therapy (HBOT) in allowing rapid tissue expansion. Additional benefits were a major increase in blood flow after the second day and continuing to the end of the experiment (one might ask why it did not occur immediately), the instant stretch back ratio when the flap is cut was lessened, the mean flap tension was less, the flap subjected to hyperbaric oxygen HBO was heavier, and the epidermal layer of the skin was thicker and held more visible vessels in subcutaneous tissue. The authors' equipment used to deliver the HBOT was an animal HBOT unit (701 Yang Park Medical Oxygen Plant, Shanghai, China) delivering 2.5 ata for 90 minutes. While Although exciting, several questions remain to be studied. Do the changes noted make a clinical difference?, are Are the parameters used by the authors for the HBOT ideal or should a dose–response curve be developed? and finally the The safety of this technique for tissue expansion in humans needs to be demonstrated.

S. H. Miller, MD

Article Index

Chapter 1: Congenital

Chapter 2: Neoplastic, Inflammatory, and Degenerative Conditions

Chapter 3: Hand and Upper Extremity

Chapter 4: Aesthetic

Chapter 5: Breast

Chapter 6: Grafts, Flaps, and Microsurgery

Chapter 7: Miscellaneous

Author Index

A

B

C

D

F

G

H

I

J

K

W

Y

Z

Kolibri 360 GmbH
Ferdinand-Jühlke-Straße 7
99095 Erfurt, Deutschland
produktsicherheit@kolibri360.de